KT-131-063

Contents

Note from the authors about the second edition

The first edition of this workbook was developed from workshop handouts used at evidence-based medicine workshops run by the Centre for Evidence-Based Medicine, Centre for General Practice, The University of Queensland. Its production was supported by the Commonwealth Department of Health and Ageing under the Primary Health Care Research Evaluation and Development Strategy.

For this second edition, we have revised the original workbook material and expanded the scope. The name of the workbook has been changed from 'Evidence-based Medicine Workbook' to 'Evidence-based Practice Workbook' to reflect the many requests that we received from users of the first edition to make this change. 'Evidence-based practice' reflects both the practical concept of evidence for what works in practice, and also the broad spectrum of health care practitioners that use the workbook.

Acknowledgements

This workbook is based on EBM workshops we have run many times in many places over the past decade. During that process, we've had help and suggestions from numerous people who we would like to thank for their feedback and ideas. Some specific folk that we would like to single out are Sandi Pirozzo (who developed many of the ideas in the appraisal sheets), Les Irwig (who gave us the ideas for the abstracts appraisal exercise), Rod Jackson and his colleagues in New Zealand (whose GATE approach to appraisal has been very influential on the methods we now use), Iain Chalmers who helped with historical examples, and the many tutors and participants in our workshops over the years. We would like to thank the Royal College of Physicians (Edinburgh) and the Wellcome Research Trust Clinical Research Facility (Edinburgh) and staff for financial and moral support in this revised and expanded version.

Accession no.
01113320
616. 0076 GLA

nch
24/7/08

Evidence-based Practice Workbook

Bridging the gap between health care research and practice

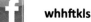

Warrington and Halton Hospitals **NHS**
NHS Foundation Trust

Knowledge
& Library Service
"Bridging the Knowledge Gap"

Alerts
Clinical
Appraisal
Literature
Information Awareness
Service Critical
Librarian Library
Management
Knowledge
Reference Practice
Evidence
Literacy

This item is to be returned on or before the last date stamped below

Mar

Professo   School

U   Australia

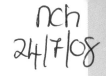 @WHHFTKLS   http://whhportal.soutron.net

                                         Tel: 01925 662128

whhftkls   Email: library@whh.nhs.uk

HALTON GENERAL HOSPITAL
EDUCATION CENTRE LIBRARY

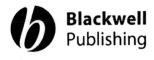
Blackwell
Publishing

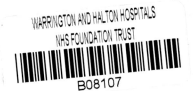
WARRINGTON AND HALTON HOSPITALS
NHS FOUNDATION TRUST

B08107

BMJ|Books

© BMJ Books, 2003
© 2007 Paul Glasziou, Chris Del Mar and Janet Salisbury
Published by Blackwell Publishing
BMJ Books is an imprint of the BMJ Publishing Group Limited, used under licence

Blackwell Publishing Inc., 350 Main Street, Malden, Massachusetts 02148-5020, USA
Blackwell Publishing Ltd, 9600 Garsington Road, Oxford OX4 2DQ, UK
Blackwell Publishing Asia Pty Ltd, 550 Swanston Street, Carlton, Victoria 3053, Australia

The right of the Author to be identified as the Author of this work has been asserted in accordance with the Copyright. Designs and Patents Act 1988.

All rights reserved. No part of this publication may be reproduced, stored in a retrieval system, or transmitted, in any form or by any means, electronic, mechanical, photocopying, recording or otherwise, as permitted by the UK Copyright, Designs and Patents Act 1988, without the prior permission of the publisher.

First published 2003
Second edition 2007

2   2008

ISBN: 978-1-4051-6728-4

A catalogue record for this title is available from the British Library

Set by Clarus Design, Canberra, Australia
Printed and bound in Singapore by COS Printers Pte Ltd
Cartoons by Ian Sharpe, Canberra, Australia

Commissioning Editor: Mary Banks
Editorial Assistant: Victoria Pittman
Development Editor: Simone Dudziak
Production Controller: Rachel Edwards

For further information on Blackwell Publishing, visit our website:
http://www.blackwellpublishing.com

The publisher's policy is to use permanent paper from mills that operate a sustainable forestry policy, and which has been manufactured from pulp processed using acid-free and elementary chlorine-free practices. Furthermore, the publisher ensures that the text paper and cover board used have met acceptable environmental accreditation standards.

Blackwell Publishing makes no representation, express or implied, that the drug dosages in this book are correct. Readers must therefore always check that any product mentioned in this publication is used in accordance with the prescribing information prepared by the manufacturers. The author and the publishers do not accept responsibility or legal liability for any errors in the text or for the misuse or misapplication of material in this book.

Introduction to this workbook

Medical practitioners, particularly GPs, are overloaded with information. They simply cannot keep up with reading all the scientific literature and other information that arrives on their desk every week. Even when they have time to read some of it, it is difficult to identify which information will be most useful in clinical practice and to recall the most up-to-date findings when they need them.

But each day doctors and health care practitioners encounter many questions that need to be answered in order to make the best decisions about patient care. This is where 'evidence-based practice' (EBP) comes in. The aim of this workbook is to introduce GPs, medical specialists, and other health care professionals to the concept of EBP and to show them simple methods to find and use the best evidence to answer their clinical questions.

The workbook is practical and interactive, and will develop your skills in:

- asking clinical questions
- searching for answers
- discriminating good from poor information and research
- using the answers to make clinical decisions.

At the end of this workbook, we hope that you will feel confident that you can find the best-quality evidence for almost any clinical question that comes your way and, with a little practice, use it to improve your clinical skills, all within a few minutes.

How to use this workbook

This workbook has been based on the evidence-based practice workshops run by the Centre for Evidence-Based Medicine and contains information and exercises to help you learn how to use EBP in your clinical practice.

The workbook is divided into three main parts:

Part 1   contains an introduction to EBP and some clinical examples to show how it can be applied.

Part 2   describes the practical application of EBP. It is subdivided into four modules, each describing an important stage in the EBP process (how to formulate a question, how to track down the best evidence, how to critically appraise the evidence and how to apply the evidence).

Part 3   includes further critical appraisal exercises on other types of clinical questions.

Part 4   contains advice on evaluating how you are going along your EBP journey as well as information on useful internet sites and other resources to help you on that journey. It also includes a Glossary of some key EBP terms used in the workbook and answers to the quizzes from earlier sections.

If you attend one of our workshops, you will find that this workbook contains all the information that will be presented during the workshop. This means that you do not need to worry about writing down a lot of notes or copying slides. Just relax and concentrate on the sessions. There are spaces in the kit for you to write down information during the interactive sessions and record the results of your EBP activities during the day.

This workbook has also been designed as a plain English resource document for anyone who is interested in learning more about EBP to study at their leisure or share with colleagues in small group training sessions.

In either case, we hope that you find it useful.

So that we can improve the workbook in future editions, please send us your suggestions (our contact details are in the 'Endpiece' at the back of the workbook).

Part 1

Introduction to evidence-based practice

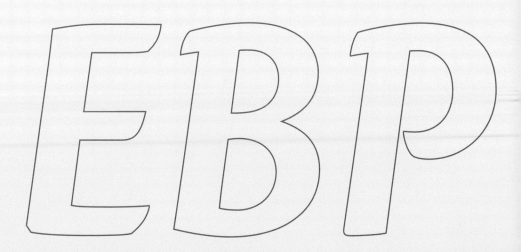

What is evidence-based practice?

Clinical practice is about making choices. Which test would be best to find out more about this condition? Which treatment would be the most effective for this patient? The answers to these questions depend on the practitioner's knowledge, skills and attitudes, the resources available and the patient's concerns, expectations and values.

In the early 1990s, David Sackett and his colleagues at McMaster University in Ontario, Canada, coined the term 'evidence-based medicine' to mean 'integrating individual clinical expertise with the best available external clinical evidence from systematic research' to achieve the best possible patient management. They have subsequently refined their definition to also take account of patient values (see box).

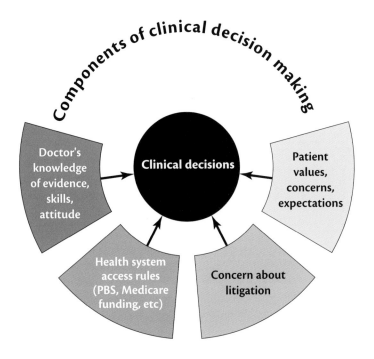

Thus, evidence-based medicine is about trying to improve the quality of the information on which health care decisions are based. It helps practitioners to avoid 'information overload' but, at the same time, to find and apply the most useful information.

The term 'evidence-based medicine', which has largely replaced the older term 'clinical epidemiology', is now often also referred to as 'evidence-based practice'. As well as being more inclusive of different areas of health care practice, the latter term highlights the important point that the 'evidence' that we are talking about is empirical evidence about what actually works or doesn't work in practice. It is not scientific evidence for a mechanism of action (such as a biochemical pathway, physiological effect or anatomical feature). Many factors affect the outcomes of clinical activities; the underlying mechanism is only one of them. Evidence-based practice (EBP) is concerned with actual clinical outcomes and is the term that we will use in this workbook.

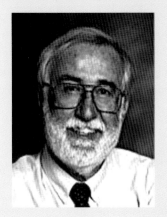

" ... the integration of **best research evidence** with **clinical expertise** and **patient values**"

– Dave Sackett

Reference:

Sackett DL, Strauss SE, Richardson WS, Rosengerg W, Haynes RB (2000). *Evidence-based Medicine: How to Practice and Teach EBM*, Churchill Livingstone, Edinburgh.

Photograph reproduced with permission.

Some essential elements of the EBP approach

1. Recognise uncertainties in clinical knowledge

2. Use research information to reduce uncertainties

3. Discriminate between strong and weak evidence

4. Quantify and communicate uncertainties with probabilities

Why do we need EBP?

Unfortunately, there is a large though variable gap between what we know from research and what we do in clinical practice. Because so much research is published — some valid and some invalid — clinicians understandably are unaware of most of it, or do not have the 'tools' to assess its quality. Researchers, on the other hand, may not understand the information needs of clinicians and often present their work in a way that is not easily accessible to busy practitioners. In 1972, British epidemiologist Archie Cochrane highlighted the fact that most treatment-related decisions were not based on a systematic review of clinical research. Rather, they were based on an ad hoc selection of information from the vast and variable quality scientific literature, on expert opinion or, worst of all, on trial and error.

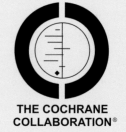

THE COCHRANE COLLABORATION®

The 'pilot' of Effective Care in Pregnancy and Childbirth then led to an international collaboration being established in response to Archie Cochrane's call for systematic, up-to-date reviews of all relevant randomised controlled trials of health care. In the early 1990s, funds were provided by the UK National Health Service to establish a Cochrane Centre in Oxford. The approach was further outlined at an international meeting organised by the New York Academy of Sciences in 1993 and at the first Cochrane Colloquium in October 1993, when 'The Cochrane Collaboration' was founded.

http://www.cochrane.org

The Cochrane logo has been reproduced with permission from The Cochrane Collaboration.

Who was Archie Cochrane?

Professor Archie Cochrane was a medical researcher in the United Kingdom who contributed to the development of epidemiology as a science. In an influential book published in 1972, *Effectiveness and Efficiency*, he drew attention to the great collective ignorance at that time about the effects of health care. He recognised that doctors did not have ready access to reliable reviews of available evidence. In a 1979 article, he said:

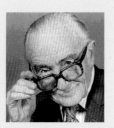

'It is surely a great criticism of our profession that we have not organised a critical summary, by speciality or subspeciality, adapted periodically, of all relevant randomised controlled trials.'

References:

Cochrane AL (1972). *Effectiveness and Efficiency: Random Reflections on Health Services*, Nuffield Provincial Hospital Trust, London (reprinted in 1989 in association with the *British Medical Journal*).

Cochrane AL (1979). 1931–1971: A critical review, with particular reference to the medical profession. In: *Medicines for the Year 2000*, Office of Health Economics, London.

Cochrane proposed that researchers and practitioners should collaborate internationally to systematically review all the best clinical trials (that is, randomised controlled trials, or RCTs), specialty by specialty. His ideas were taken up during the 1980s by Iain Chalmers who persuaded colleagues to join him and make care during pregnancy and childbirth the first area of clinical practice to be reviewed in this way. Systematic reviews of RCTs of different aspects of obstetric care soon showed some anomalies between the clinical trial evidence and established practice. This highlighted the gaps that existed between research and clinical practice and started to convince some doctors of the benefits of an evidence-based approach to bridge this gap.

This work has been continued though The Cochrane Collaboration (see box), which publishes systematic reviews of RCTs electronically in the Cochrane Database of Systematic Reviews, within The Cochrane Library. Access to The Cochrane Library is available free online in many countries.

Go to **http://www.cochrane.org** and follow the prompts for The Cochrane Library.

CORTICOSTEROIDS FOR PRETERM BIRTH

1972

An RCT was published that showed improved outcomes for preterm babies when mothers were given a short course of corticosteroids before the birth.

1972–89

Six more RCTs were published, all confirming the 1972 findings.

During this time, most obstetricians were still unaware that corticosteroid treatment was effective and so did not treat women who were about to have a preterm birth with corticosteroids.

1989

The first systematic review of corticosteroid treatment was published.

1989–91

Seven more studies were published.

Conclusion

Corticosteroid treatment reduces the odds of babies dying from complications of immaturity by 30 to 50%, but thousands of babies have died or suffered unnecessarily since 1972 because doctors did not know about the effectiveness of the treatment shown in the 1972 trial, and were misled by subsequent smaller trials until these were combined ('meta-analysed').

The flecainide story

The history of the use of the drug flecainide to treat heart attacks in the United States in the 1980s is a dramatic example of the gap between research and clinical practice, and of the reliance on evidence of a mechanism rather than an outcome. In 1979, the developer of the defibrillator, Bernard Lown, pointed out in an address to the American College of Cardiology that one of the biggest causes of death was heart attack, particularly among young and middle-aged men (20–64-year-olds). People had a heart attack, developed arrhythmia and died from the arrhythmia. He suggested that a 'safe and long-acting antiarrhythmic drug that protects against ventricular fibrillation' would save millions of lives.

In response to this challenge, a paper was published in the *New England Journal of Medicine* introducing a new drug called flecainide — a local anesthetic derivative that suppresses arrhythmia. The paper described a study in which patients who had just had heart attacks were randomly assigned to groups to receive either a placebo or flecainide and were then switched from one group to the other (a cross-over trial). The researchers counted the number of premature ventricular contractions (PVCs) as a measure of arrhythmias. The patients on flecainide had fewer PVCs than the patients on placebo. When the flecainide patients were 'crossed over' to the placebo treatment, the PVCs increased again.

Suppression of arrhythmias in nine patients
(Each line represents one patient)

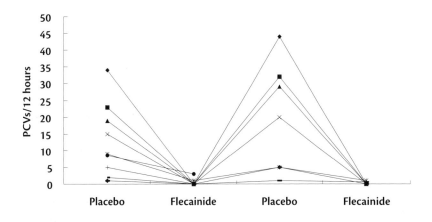

The conclusion was straightforward: flecainide reduces arrhythmias, arrhythmias cause heart attacks (the mechanism); therefore, people who have had heart attacks should be given flecainide. After the results were published, flecainide was approved by the United States Food and Drug Administration and became fairly standard treatment for heart attack in the United States (although it did not catch on in Europe or Australia).

Almost immediately after the first trials were complete, however, other researchers had started gathering information on the survival of the patients (the outcome) instead of the PVC rate (the mechanism). This showed that over the 18 months following treatment, more than 10% of people who were given flecainide died, which was double the rate of deaths among a placebo group. In other words, despite a perfectly good mechanism for the usefulness of flecainide (it reduces arrhythmias), the drug was clearly toxic and, overall, did more harm than good.

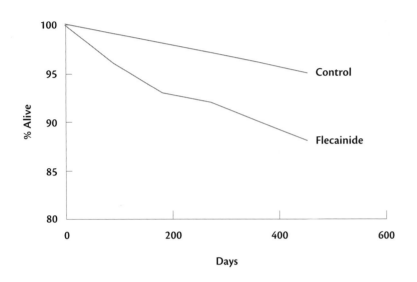

Cardiac arrhythmia suppression trial

Key issues

Overall, the flecainide story raises two important issues:

- We need a better way to find information, even when we do not know that we need it. In other words, up-to-date, good-quality research findings need to be available to all medical practitioners on a routine basis.

- The type of research is important. We must move away from a traditional mechanistic approach and look for empirical evidence of effectiveness using a clinically relevant outcome (such as survival, improved quality of life).

Unfortunately, because the initial studies had been widely published in medical texts, it was a long time before doctors caught up with the subsequent data showing poor outcomes, which did not attract as much attention. Meanwhile, by 1989, about 200,000 people were being treated with flecainide in the United States. Based on the trial evidence, this would have caused tens of thousands of additional heart attack deaths due to the use of flecainide. Although there was published information, doctors were systematically killing people with flecainide because they did not know about the good-quality outcome-based research.

What does the flecainide example tell us?

In the flecainide example, the initial research was widely disseminated because it was based on a traditional mechanistic approach to medicine, and because it offered a 'cure'. The subsequent outcomes research may not have been widely disseminated because it was counterintuitive and negative in terms of a potential treatment. Doctors continued to prescribe flecainide because they believed that it worked. They did not know that they needed to look for additional information.

References:

Anderson JL, Stewart JR, Perry BA et al (1981). Oral flecainide acetate for the treatment of ventricular arrhythmias. *New England Journal of Medicine* 305:473–477.

Echt DS, Liebson PR, Mitchell LB et al (1991). Mortality and morbidity in patients receiving ecainide, flecainide, or placebo. The Cardiac Arrhythmia Suppression Trial. *New England Journal of Medicine* 324:781–788.

Moore TJ (1995). *Deadly Medicine*, Simon and Schuster, New York.

So much evidence, so little time

Doctors need to be linked to the medical research literature in a way that allows them to routinely obtain up-to-date, outcomes-based information. However, most medical practitioners, particularly GPs, are overloaded with information. Unsolicited information received though the mail alone can amount to kilograms per month and most of it ends up in the bin.

The total number of RCTs published has increased exponentially since the 1940s. A total of 20,000 trials are published each year (with more than 400,000 trials in total). In 2005, approximately 55 new trials were published every day. Therefore, to keep up to date with RCTs alone, a GP would have to read more than one study report every half hour, day and night. In addition to RCTs, in 2005, about 1800 papers were also indexed daily on MEDLINE from a total of probably 5000 journal articles published each day.

The amount of medical research

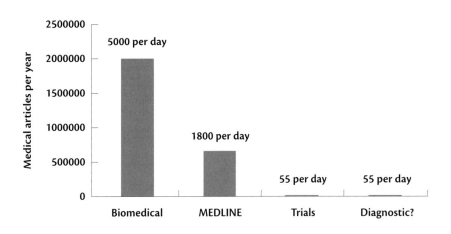

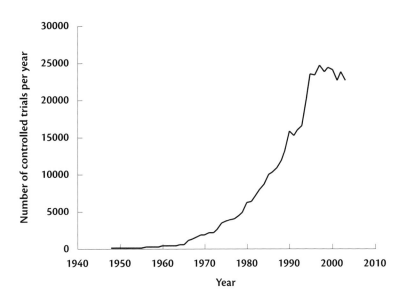

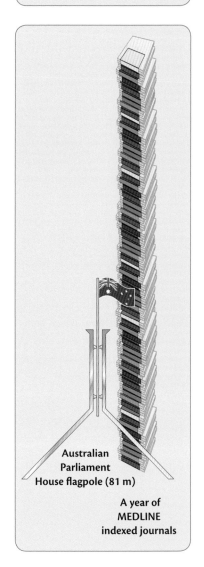

Australian
Parliament
House flagpole (81 m)

**A year of
MEDLINE
indexed journals**

'Kill as few patients as possible'

A book by physician and medical humorist Oscar London, called *Kill as Few Patients as Possible*, gives a set of 'rules' for clinical practice.

Rule 31 offers some advice on how to keep up to date with medical research:

'Review the world literature fortnightly'

Reference:

London O (1987). *Kill as Few Patients as Possible: And 56 Other Essays on How to Be the World's Best Doctor*, Edition 2, Ten Speed Press, Berkeley, California, USA.

At best, most GPs give a selective sample of the literature a cursory review, but very little is properly assessed and almost none influences what they do in practice.

Doctors may feel guilty, anxious or inadequate because of this (see box on the JASPA criteria), but it is not their fault — there is just too much information. There needs to be a better way.

JASPA criteria
(journal-associated score of personal angst)

Can you answer these five simple questions:

J   Are you ambivalent about renewing your **journal** subscriptions?

A   Do you feel **anger** towards particular authors?

S   Do you use journals to help you **sleep**?

P   Are you surrounded by piles of **periodicals**?

A   Do you feel **anxious** when another one comes through the letterbox?

Score (Yes = 1; No = 0):
0   anyone who scores zero is probably a liar!
1–3   normal range
>3   sick, at risk for 'polythenia gravis' and related conditions

Reference:

Modified from 'Polythenia gravis: the downside of evidence-based medicine.' *British Medical Journal* (1995) 311:1666–1668.

How do doctors try to overcome information overload?

Write down some education activities that you and your organisation engage in and how much time you spend on them.

Rank your activities from most to least time.

Then for your top activities/sources, ask yourself the following questions: Where do questions come from? How is the information selected? Is the information appraised (or do you appraise it)?

Your education activities	How much time do you spend on each?	Rank

You have probably included a selection of activities including attending lectures and conferences, reading journals and 'throwaways', textbooks and clinical practice guidelines, electronic searching, clinical attachments, and small-group learning.

You may also have included talking to colleagues or specialists. But everyone has the same problem of keeping up to date and your colleagues may be out of date or just plain wrong. If they have got the information from somewhere else, you need to know where they got it so that you can check how good it is. Textbooks are always about 5–10 years out of date.

Faced with all the alternatives, how do you actually choose what to do in your continuing education time? If you are honest, your choice probably depends on what you are already most interested in rather than what you don't know about.

Continuing medical education (CME) has been a mainstay of doctors' professional development but no-one has ever shown that it works. When doctors choose their courses, they choose things that they think they need to know about. But as we have seen, the most important information is what they don't know they need! In other words, we need a system to tell us we need to know something.

In a trial of CME, a random sample of GPs were asked to rank 18 selected conditions into either a 'high preference' set for which they wanted to receive CME, or a 'low preference set' for which they did not want further education. Physicians with similar rankings were paired and randomised to either:

- a control group, whose CME was postponed for 18 months; or

- an experimental group, who received CME at once for their high preference topics and were provided with training materials for their low preference topics, which they were asked to promise to study.

The outcomes were measured in terms of the quality of clinical care (QOC) provided by each of the physicians before and after CME (determined from clinical records). The results showed that although the knowledge of the physicians in the experimental group rose after their CME, the effects on QOC were disappointing with a similar (small) increase in QOC for both the experimental and control groups for their high preference conditions.

By contrast, for low preference conditions, QOC rose significantly for the experimental physicians but fell for the control group.

A review of didactic CME by Davis et al (1999) also concluded that formal sessions are not effective in changing physician performance.

Conclusions of CME trial

1. If you want CME on a topic, you don't need it.

2. CME on a topic only works when you don't want it.

3. CME does not cause general improvements in the quality of care.

References:

Sibley JC, Sackett DL, Neufeld V et al (1982). A randomised trial of continuing medical education. *New England Journal of Medicine* 306:511–515.

Davis D, O'Brien MA, Freemantle N et al (1999). Impact of formal continuing medical education: do conferences, workshops, rounds, and other traditional continuing education activities change physician behavior or health care outcomes? *JAMA* 282(9):867–874.

Overall, as we have seen, there is too much information but we still need it. The quality of most of this information is very poor: most published information is irrelevant and/or the methods are not good. Finding the high-quality evidence is like trying to sip pure water from a hose pumping dirty water, or looking for 'rare pearls'.

High-quality/relevant data — pearls

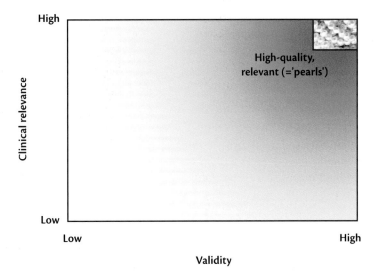

How many questions can doctors answer each day?

Many questions arise every day as a result of seeing people in clinical practice. Two papers have been published on this: one of interns in a hospital setting and one of GPs. In both cases, the researchers asked the doctors to note every time a question arose and what information they needed.

The study of 100 GPs showed that they each wrote down about 10 questions over a 2.5-day period. The GPs tried to find answers for about half of these. The most critical factor influencing which questions they followed up was how long they thought it would take to get an answer. If the doctor thought the answer would be available in less than a couple of minutes, they were prepared to look for it. If they thought it would take longer, they would not bother. Only two questions in the whole study (ie 2/1000) were followed up using a proper electronic search.

Doctors' information needs

Study 1 (interns)

- 64 residents in 2 hospitals were interviewed after 401 consultations
- They asked an average of 280 questions (2 questions for every 3 patients seen)
- At interview two weeks later, they had followed up an answer for only 80 questions (29%)
- Other questions were not pursued:
  - because of lack of time, or
  - because they forgot the question
- Sources of answers to questions were:
  - textbooks (31%)
  - articles (21%)
  - consultants (17%)

Study 2 (GPs)

- 103 GPs in Iowa collected questions over 2.5 days
- A total of 1101 questions were collected
- Pursued answers in 702 (64%)
- Spent less than 2 minutes pursuing an answer using readily available print and human resources
- Only 2 questions (0.2%) led to a formal literature search

References:

Green ML, Ciampi MA and Ellis PJ (2000). Residents' medical information needs in clinic: are they being met? *Americal Journal of Medicine* 109:218–233.

Ely JW, Osheroff JA, Ebell MH et al (1999). Analysis of questions asked by family doctors regarding patient care. *British Medical Journal* 319: 358–361.

Information gathering

There are two ways in which we all get information:

- just in case — in an ad hoc way from the vast amount of information that crosses our desk or arrives in our inbox daily ('push'), or

- just in time — in a targeted way, by seeking out information in response to a specific question ('pull').

'Push' new relevant and valid results

For EBP, the best sources for the 'push' approach to improving knowledge ('just-in-case' learning) are where the 'pearls' have already been selected from the rest of the lower-quality literature. Some good sources of information where this has been done include:

Evidence-Based Medicine — one of several 'evidence-based' journals that scan more than 100 journals for valid articles and then have clinicians around the world assess their clinical relevance and importance to clinical practice. The EBM journal is published every two months and has no original articles, but gives a condensed version of the original paper.

The journal is also available on the internet at:
http://www.evidence-basedmedicine.com

Clinical Evidence — a compendium of evidence-based literature searches. It is updated and published every 6 months as a book and CD. Information is arranged by specialty and just states the best existing evidence for an intervention. If there is no evidence, it says so. It does not include opinions or consensus guidelines. The editors decide what questions are relevant but the book is based on what doctors need. Doctors can look up information when they need it (the 'pull' method of obtaining information).

Clinical Evidence is available on the internet at:
http://www.clinicalevidence.com

'Pull' answers in less than 2 minutes

In this workbook, we will focus on learning how to formulate questions and 'pull' answers out of the literature in less than 2 minutes! This is sometimes called 'just-in-time' learning.

In the next few pages we will look at some case studies where EBP methods were used.

Balance your information: 'push' and 'pull'

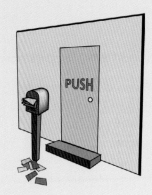

'Push' (or 'just-in-case' learning) is when we receive information from a variety of sources and on a variety of topics and extract what we think we need for our practice.

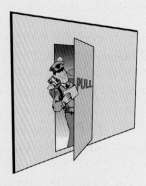

'Pull' (or 'just-in-time' learning) is when we deliberately seek information to answer a specific question.

Some evidence-based cases

In this section we will discuss several case studies that show how EBP can help in a range of clinical situations. You can then think of a clinical question of your own and we will try to answer it.

Case study 1: persistent cough

A 58-year-old who was visiting her GP about another matter said, as an aside, 'Can you do anything about a cough?' She had had a persistent cough for 20 years with various treatments but no cure. She had been referred twice to physicians.

The GP searched PubMed (the web-based version of MEDLINE) using 'Clinical Queries', which is a category of PubMed designed for clinicians (see pages 56–58). The search for persistent cough revealed that the most common causes are:

- postnasal drip
- asthma
- chronic bronchitis.

The GP thought the cough was most likely to be due to asthma, and prescribed appropriate first-line treatment. The patient thought she had already tried that treatment and that it did not work but tried it again anyway, without success. However, the search also showed that gastro-oesophageal reflux is a less common but possible cause of persistent cough (10% of cases), which the GP had not known before. The GP therefore recommended the patient to take antacids at night and raise the head of her bed. After one week, her cough disappeared for the first time in 20 years and has not come back since.

How did EBP help?

This case raises interesting questions of what doctors 'should' know. It was written up in the BMJ and published as an example of how EBP can help GPs. However, some physicians wrote in saying that 'everyone should know' that gastro-oesophageal reflux was a possible cause of cough. The author replied that although respiratory physicians might know this information, GPs did not necessarily know it. An anaesthetist wrote in to say that after reading the article he had been treated for gastro-oesophageal reflux, which had cured a cough he had had for 30 years!

Conclusion: EBP can help you find the information you need, whether or not you 'should' already know it.

Reference:

Glasziou P (1998). Evidence based case report: Twenty year cough in a non-smoker. *British Medical Journal* 316:1660–1661.

Case study 2: dog bite

A patient came to the clinic with a fresh dog bite. It looked clean and the GP and patient wondered whether it was necessary to give prophylactic antibiotics. The GP searched MEDLINE and found a meta-analysis indicating that the average infection rate for dog bites was 14% and that antibiotics halved this risk. In other words:

- for every 100 people with dog bites, treatment with antibiotics will save 7 from becoming infected; or

- treating 14 people with dog bites will prevent one infection.

The second number (14) is called the 'number needed to treat' (NNT).

The GP explained these figures to the patient, along with the possible consequences of an infection, and the patient decided not to take antibiotics. On follow-up, it was found that he did not get infected.

How did EBP help?

In this case, EBP helped because the empirical data were easy for the patient to understand and he could participate in the clinical decision. As the culture of health care changes further towards consumer participation in health care decision making, patients will demand this type of information.

Reference:

Cummings P (1994). Antibiotics to prevent infection in patients with dog bite wounds: a meta-analysis of randomized trials. *Annals of Emergency Medicine* 23:535–540.

Empirical measures of outcomes

Outcomes are commonly measured as absolute risk reduction (ARR), relative risks (RR) and number needed to treat (NNT).

The risk of infection after dog bite with no antibiotics
= 14% (0.14)

The risk of infection after dog bite with antibiotics
= 7% (0.07)

The ARR for antibiotic treatment
= 14 − 7 = 7%
(That is, 7 people in every 100 treated will be saved from infection.)

NNT = 100/7
= 14
(That is, you would need to treat 14 dog bite patients with antibiotics to prevent 1 infection.)

RR of infection with antibiotics compared to without antibiotics
= 0.07/0.14
= 0.5 (50%)

NOTE: It is best to quote the ARR or NNT in discussions with patients. The RR is harder to put into context because it is independent of the frequency of the 'problem' (the 'event rate'), in this case, the rate at which people with dog bites get infected. Further information on these measures is given in EBP Step 3 (Rapid critical appraisal).

Case study 3: microscopic blood in the urine

One of us, then a healthy 47-year-old male, was acting as a patient in a medical exam. The students accurately found microscopic traces of blood in his urine. He went to his GP and was retested a month later. The blood was still there. The GP suggested conventional investigation: an ultrasound and cystoscopy. It was time to search the literature for evidence of the effectiveness of these procedures.

He searched for a cohort study of 40–50-year-olds with haematuria with long-term follow-up and for RCTs of screening for haematuria. He used the search categories 'prognosis' and 'specificity' and the search terms 'haematuria OR hematuria'. He got 300 hits. Two papers were very relevant (see box).

Therefore, he concluded that blood in urine is not a good indicator of bladder cancer and did not have the cystoscopy test.

How did EBP help?

The lesson from this case concerns the practical versus the empirical. Doctors tend to think along the lines of:

> Blood does not belong in the urine so it must be coming from somewhere. It could be coming from a potentially serious cause, such as bladder cancer.

Empirical questions, on the other hand, ask about outcomes — in this case, whether conventional investigation leads to better health outcomes. Here, the evidence (surprisingly) showed that such investigation provides no benefit, because microscopic haematuria seems to be no more prevalent among those who later develop urological cancer than those who do not. Once again, being empirical and quantitative allows patients to participate much more fully in clinical decisions.

Study 1

10,000 men were screened. About 250 (2.5%) had haematuria. These men were asked to visit their GP and about 150 (60%) did so. Of those, only three had a serious problem. Of these:

- 2 had bladder cancer
- 1 had reflux nephropathy.

This shows that there is about a 1 in 50 chance of having a serious disease.

Study 2

As part of a personal health appraisal, 20,000 men were given a urine test. Follow-up studies of the men who were positive for haematuria found three cancers per year, or 1.5 cancers per 1000 person-years. However, the people who did not have haematuria were also followed up and the rate of cancer for these people was exactly the same as for the people with haematuria.

EBP can help to reduce litigation

This case raises the issue of possible litigation. What if the patient is not tested and later develops a serious disease? However, because EBP improves communication between doctors and patients and allows patients to share decision making, it protects doctors from litigation (because most litigation happens when there is a breakdown in communication). EBP analyses have already been used in the courts and have been well accepted. Such empirical evidence has saved doctors from trouble when opinion may have damned them.

Reference:

Del Mar C (2000). Asymptomatic haematuria ... in the doctor. *British Medical Journal* 320:165–166.

Summary of case studies

The case studies show that EBP has several advantages.

- Medical practitioners, especially GPs, can't know everything. EBP helps doctors keep up to date across a very wide spectrum of information.

- MEDLINE and similar databases have several advantages. For medical practitioners, they are a way of finding good-quality, up-to-date information that is less likely to be biased than information obtained from other sources (such as from company representatives).

- Because the search is based on questions rather than possible answers, doctors can find information without needing to have known about it before. In other words, they can find information that they do not initially know they need, but which, as we have seen, is vitally important for good clinical practice.

- The evidence can be used to quantify outcomes (empirical evidence). This allows people to assess the likelihood of benefiting from a particular treatment or activity rather than just considering the underlying mechanism.

- Patients like this empirical approach because it is easier to understand and allows them to share in decision making. This reduces the chances of future litigation.

- Electronic searching can reveal other useful information that may benefit the patient.

The steps in evidence-based practice

Part 2 of this workbook looks at the four basic steps involved in EBP (see box).

First we will work out how to turn your day-to-day questions into a form that can be used to search the medical literature in less than two minutes. Next we will find out how to use PubMed (MEDLINE), The Cochrane Library and other resources to search electronically for the information we need. After this, we will find out how to assess the articles we find in the searches, work out what the results mean and assess how they can be applied to individual patients. Part 3 includes further information on assessing different types of clinical studies and Part 4 includes reflections on the process of EBP and supplies some further information and readings, plus a Glossary and answers to selected questions.

Steps in EBP

1. Formulate an answerable question.

2. Track down the best evidence of outcomes.

3. Critically appraise the evidence (to find out how good it is and what it means).

4. Apply the evidence (integrate the results with clinical expertise and patient values).

As an additional 'meta-step', it is important to keeping asking how we are doing (so that we can improve next time).

Notes

Part 2

The steps in evidence-based practice

EBP

EBP Step 1: Formulate an answerable question

First principle

First, you must admit that you don't know. As we have already seen, it is impossible to know everything. Evidence-based practice (EBP) gives you a method to find answers to research answerable questions that arise in daily clinical work.

On the next page, jot down some clinical questions or problems that have occurred to you lately. Don't think too hard; just write down the last few things that have cropped up in your work or family life.

Steps in EBP

1. Formulate an answerable question.

2. Track down the best evidence of outcomes available.

3. Critically appraise the evidence (find out how good it is and what it means).

4. Apply the evidence (integrate the results with clinical expertise and patient values).

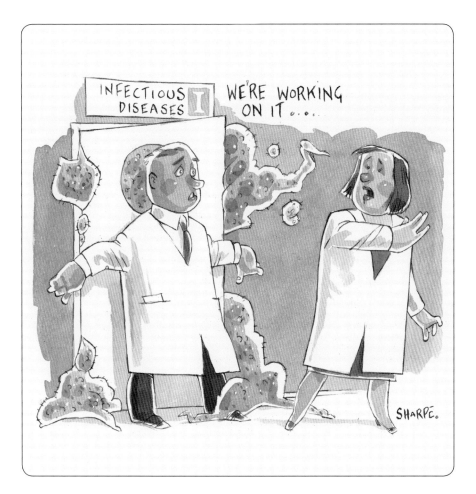

Your clinical questions:

Different types of clinical question

Compare your list of questions with others in your class or group. What types of questions do you have? The following classification covers the main types of questions that crop up in health care practice.

Question	Question type	Description
What should I do about this condition or problem?	Intervention	By far the most common type of clinical question is about how to treat a disease or condition, or how to alleviate other health care problems. We refer to such actions as 'interventions'.
What causes the problem?	Aetiology and risk factors	We often would like to know the cause of health care problems, such as whether cigarette smoking causes lung cancer, or being overweight increases the risk of heart disease.
Does this person have the condition or problem?	Diagnosis	In order to treat a person, it is first important to correctly determine what the health care condition or problem is. Because most detection methods are not 100% accurate, questions of diagnosis often arise, related to the accuracy of available tests.
Who will get the condition or problem?	Prognosis and prediction	A necessary precursor to treatment is to know the likelihood that a person will develop a particular condition or problem so as to target preventative actions. For example, a patient's risk of stroke or deep vein thrombosis, or young children's risk of learning difficulties.
How common is the problem?	Frequency and rate	It is often important to know the prevalence (frequency) or incidence (rate) of a health care problem in the population. For example, the frequency of a particular birth defect in mothers of a particular age or genetic background, or the incidence of an infectious disease during summer or winter.
What are the types of problems?	Phenomena or thoughts	Finally, some questions relate to more general issues, such as the concerns of parents about vaccination of their children, or the barriers to lifestyle change such as healthy eating.

The 'PICO' principle

Our questions are often only partly formulated, which makes finding answers in the medical literature a challenge. Dissecting the question into its component parts and restructuring it so that it is easy to find the answers is an essential first step in EBP. Most questions can be divided into four components:

Population and clinical problem	This shows who the relevant people are in relation to the clinical problem that you have in mind.
Intervention (or indicator or index text)*	This shows the management strategy, exposure or test that that you want to find out about in relation to the clinical problem. This might be:
	• a procedure, such as a drug treatment, surgery or diet (**intervention**)
	• exposure to an environmental chemical or other hazard, a physical feature (such as being overweight), or a factor that might affect a health outcome (**indicator**)
	• a diagnostic test, such as a blood test or brain scan (**index test**).
Comparator	This shows an alternative or control strategy, exposure or test for comparison with the one you are interested in.
Outcome	This shows:
	• what are you most concerned about happening (or stopping happening) AND/OR
	• what the patient is most concerned about.

*   In the remainder of this workbook, we have used these specific terms where possible for different types of questions. In other places, 'Intervention' is used as a generic term.

We call these four parts of a clinical question 'PICO' (pronounced 'pee-co'), which makes them easy to remember. A timeframe (T) is usually implicit in every question, but it is sometimes useful to add this component explicitly (ie PICOT).

In the following pages, we will see how to use the PICO principle for each type of clinical question. It is important to structure your questions using these components if possible, although, as we will see, you may not need to use all the components for every type of question.

Remember the PICO principle

 Population/problem

 Intervention

 Comparator/control

 Outcome

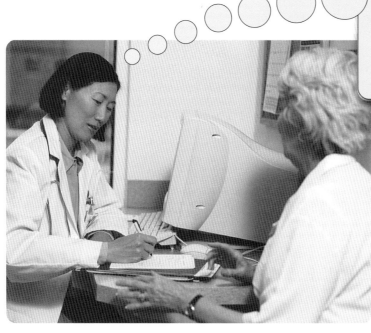

Interventions

Interventions cover a wide range of activities from drug treatments and other clinical therapies, to lifestyle changes (for example, diet or exercise) and social activities (such as counselling or education programs). Interventions can include individual patient care or population health activities (for example, screening for diseases such as cervical or prostate cancer). The critical question in every case is whether the intervention actually improves things for the individual or population concerned.

Example 1

Jean is a 55-year-old woman who quite often crosses the Atlantic to visit her elderly mother. She tends to get swollen legs on these flights and is worried about her risk of developing deep vein thrombosis (DVT), because she has read quite a bit about this in the newspapers lately. She asks you if she should wear elastic stockings on her next trip to reduce her risk of this.

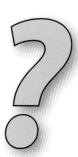

To convert this to an answerable question, use the PICO method as follows:

P *Population/problem* = passengers on long-haul flights

I *Intervention* = wearing elastic compression stockings

C *Comparator/control* = no elastic stockings

O *Outcome* = development of DVT

Question:

'In passengers on long-haul flights, does wearing elastic compression stockings, compared with not wearing elastic stockings, prevent DVT?'

Example 2

Jeff, a smoker of more than 30 years, has come to see you about something unrelated. You ask him if he is interested in stopping smoking. He tells you he has tried to quit smoking unsuccessfully in the past. A friend of his, however, successfully quit with acupuncture. Should he try it? Other interventions you know about are nicotine replacement therapy and antidepressants.

Develop a clinical research question using PICO:

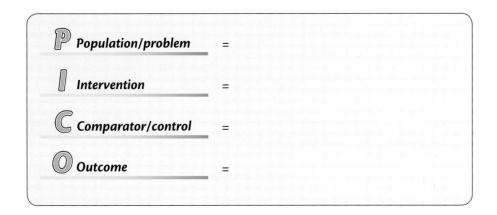

P *Population/problem* =

I *Intervention* =

C *Comparator/control* =

O *Outcome* =

Question:

_____

_____

_____

Example 3

At a routine immunisation visit, Lisa, the mother of a six-month-old, tells you
that her baby suffered a nasty local reaction after her previous immunisation.
Lisa is very concerned that the same thing may happen again this time.
Recently, a colleague told you that needle length can affect local reactions to
immunisation in young children but you can't remember the precise details.

Develop a clinical research question using PICO to help you find the
information you need:

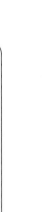

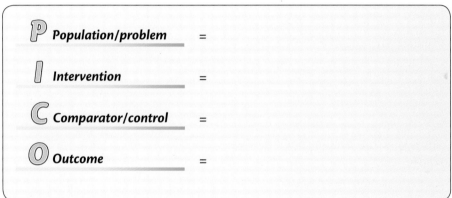

Question:

_____

_____

_____

_____

_____

Answers to these question exercises are in the 'Answers' section in Part 4 of this workbook.

Aetiology and risk factors

Questions of *aetiology and risk factors* are about what causes a disease or health condition. These are the reverse of intervention questions because they deal with harmful outcomes of an activity or exposure. Such questions commonly arise in relation to public health issues, such as whether eating certain foods increases the risk of heart disease, or being exposed to an environmental chemical increases the risk of cancer, and so on.

Example 1

George has come to your surgery to discuss the possibility of getting a vasectomy. He says he has heard something about vasectomy causing an increase in testicular cancer later in life. You know that the risk of this is very low but want to give him a more precise answer.

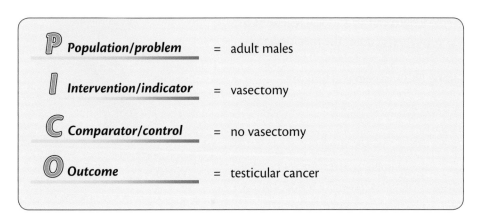

P	**Population/problem**	=	adult males
I	**Intervention/indicator**	=	vasectomy
C	**Comparator/control**	=	no vasectomy
O	**Outcome**	=	testicular cancer

Question:

'In men, does having a vasectomy (compared with not having one), increase the risk of getting testicular cancer in the future?'

Example 2

Susan is expecting her first baby in two months. She has been reading about the potential benefits and harms of giving newborn babies vitamin K injections. She is alarmed by reports that vitamin K injections in newborn babies may cause childhood leukaemia. She asks you if this is true and, if so, what the risk for her baby will be.

Develop a clinical research question using PICO to help answer Susan's question:

P Population/problem	=
I Intervention/indicator	=
C Comparator/control	=
O Outcome	=

Question:

_____

_____

_____

Diagnosis

Diagnosis questions are concerned with how accurate a diagnostic test is in various patient groups and in comparison with other available tests. Measures of test accuracy include its sensitivity, specificity, and positive and negative predictive value.

Example 1

Julie is pregnant for the second time. She had her first baby when she was 33 and had amniocentesis to find out if the baby had Down syndrome. The test was negative but it was not a good experience, because she did not get the result until she was 18 weeks pregnant. She is now 35 and 1 month pregnant, and asks if she can have a test that would give her an earlier result. The local hospital offers serum biochemistry plus nuchal translucency ultrasound screening as a first trimester test for Down syndrome. You wonder if this combination of tests is as reliable as conventional amniocentesis.

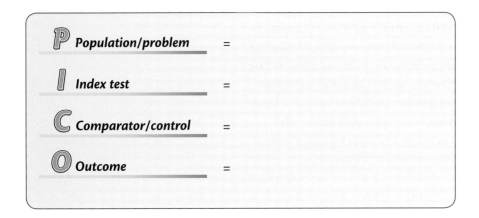

	P Population/problem	=	pregnant women (first trimester)
	I Index test	=	nuchal translucency ultrasound screening plus serum biochemistry
	C Comparator/control	=	conventional amniocentesis
	O Outcome	=	accurate diagnosis (measured by sensitivity and specificity of Down syndrome (trisomy 21))

Question:

'For pregnant women, is nuchal translucency ultrasound screening plus serum biochemistry testing in the first trimester as accurate (ie with equal or better sensitivity and specificity) as conventional amniocentesis for diagnosing Down syndrome?'

Example 2

As part of your clinic's assessment of elderly patients, there is a hearing check. Over a tea-room discussion, it turns out that some people simply ask, while others use a tuning fork, but you claim that a simple whispered voice test is very accurate. Challenged to back this up with evidence, you promise to do a literature search before tomorrow's meeting.

Develop a clinical research question using PICO to help you with your literature research:

P Population/problem	=
I Index test	=
C Comparator/control	=
O Outcome	=

Question:

Prognosis (prediction)

Prognosis (prediction) questions are concerned with how likely an outcome is for a population with certain characteristics (risk factors), such as the likelihood that a man who is experiencing atypical chest pains will suffer further heart failure or sudden death within the next few days, or the predicted morbidity and mortality for a person diagnosed with colon cancer.

Example 1

Childhood seizures are common and frightening for the parents, and the decision to initiate prophylactic treatment after a first fit is a difficult one. To help parents make their decision, you need to explain the risk of further occurrences following a single seizure of unknown cause.

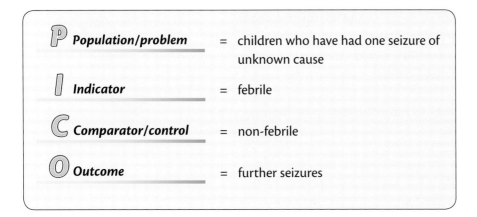

P *Population/problem*	=	children who have had one seizure of unknown cause
I *Indicator*	=	febrile
C *Comparator/control*	=	non-febrile
O *Outcome*	=	further seizures

Question:

'In children who have had one seizure of unknown cause (either associated with a fever or not), what is the long-term risk of further seizures?'

However, note that many prognosis questions begin with the population or problem and outcome only (ie only consist of a 'P' and an 'O'). This is because most prognosis studies relate to fairly broad populations rather than 'drilling' down to compare subgroups. For the above example, the question could therefore also be expressed as:

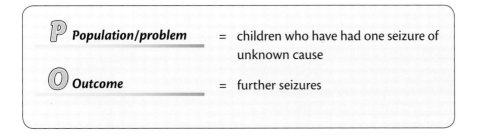

P *Population/problem*	=	children who have had one seizure of unknown cause
O *Outcome*	=	further seizures

Question:

'In children who have had one seizure of unknown cause, what is the long-term risk of further seizures?'

Framing the question this way (PO only) would provide enough information to find studies relevant to this issue, including any that do compare children who have had a previous seizure with those who have not. Beyond this, we may want to refine the prognosis based on a number of features (or indicators), such as whether the child was febrile, the duration of seizure, the age of the child. The PO gives us an initial base, which the PICO can refine.

Example 2

Mr Thomas, who is 58 years old, has correctly diagnosed his inguinal lump as a hernia. He visits you for confirmation of his diagnosis and information about the consequences. You mention the possibility of strangulation, and the man asks: 'How likely is that?' You reply 'pretty unlikely' (which is as much as you know at the time) but say that you will try to find out more precisely.

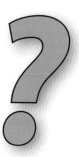

Develop a clinical research question using PICO to help you give Mr Thomas more precise details about his prognosis:

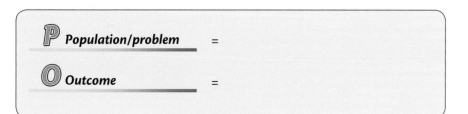

P **Population/problem** =

O **Outcome** =

Question:

_____

_____

Frequency or rate

Questions of frequency (prevalence) are about how many people in the population have a disease or health problem, such as what is the frequency of hearing problems in infants or the prevalence of Alzheimer's disease in over 70-year-olds. If the question also includes a time period, such as for cases of influenza in winter versus summer, it becomes a question of rate (incidence).

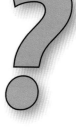

In the same way as we have already seen for prognosis questions, as frequency and rate questions relate to whole populations, they can usually be framed in terms of the 'P' and 'O' components only.

Example 1

Mabel is a six-week-old baby at her routine follow-up. She was born prematurely at 35 weeks. Her parents ask about her chances of developing hearing problems, as friends of theirs had a premature baby with deafness that was detected late.

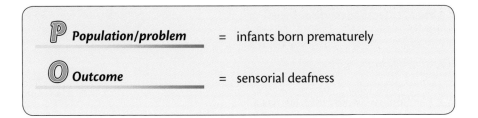

P *Population/problem*	=	infants born prematurely
O *Outcome*	=	sensorial deafness

Question:

'In infants born prematurely, what is the frequency of sensorial deafness?'

Example 2

Mrs Smith has acute lower back pain. She has never had such pain before and is convinced that it must be caused by something really serious. You take a history and examine her but find no indicators of a more serious condition. You reassure her that the majority of acute low back pain is not serious, but she is still not convinced.

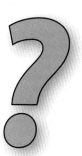

Develop a clinical research question using PICO to help reassure Mrs Smith:

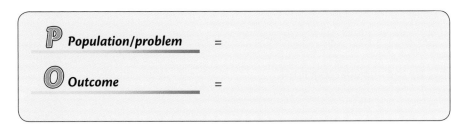

P *Population/problem*	=	
O *Outcome*	=	

Question:

Phenomena

Questions about phenomena or thoughts can relate to any aspects of clinical practice, such as physical examination, taking a health history, or barriers to successful participation in health care.

Once again, such questions usually only involve a population (P) and an outcome (O), and the outcome is often a broad category (eg ideas, beliefs or concerns).

Example 1

Mary is a mother who is concerned about her three-year-old child. He has a fever. After you have examined him, you conclude that he probably has a viral infection. Mary asks, 'But what if he has a fever again during the night, doctor?' You want to understand her principal underlying concerns so that you can reassure her.

Develop a clinical research question using PICO to help you answer this question:

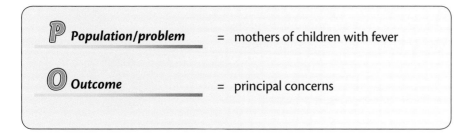

P	Population/problem	= mothers of children with fever
O	Outcome	= principal concerns

Question:

'For mothers of children with a fever, what are the principal concerns?'

Example 2

When you are writing a repeat prescription for a patient, they tell you they remember to take their tablets by setting an alarm on their mobile phone. You start to wonder about what methods patients have used to help them remember medications.

Develop a clinical research question using PICO to help you answer this question:

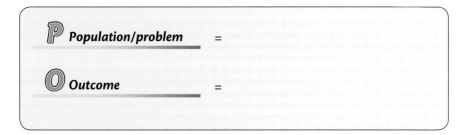

P	Population/problem	=
O	Outcome	=

Your own questions

Write here the clinical issue that you wrote down earlier (page 22):

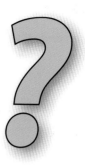

_____

_____

_____

Identify what sort of question it is (circle):

intervention   aetiology/   diagnosis   prognosis/   frequency/   phenomenon
            risk   prediction   rate

Now build up a research question using P I C O

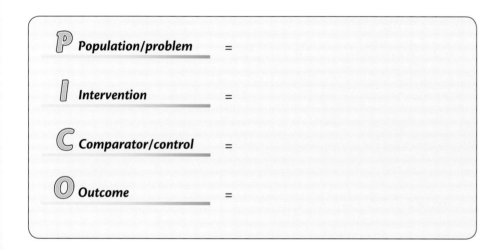

Question:

_____

_____

_____

Your own questions

Write a second clinical issue that interests you:

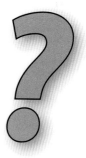

_____

_____

_____

Identify what sort of question it is (circle):

intervention   aetiology/   diagnosis   prognosis/   frequency/   phenomenon
                risk   prediction   rate

Now build up a research question using P I C O

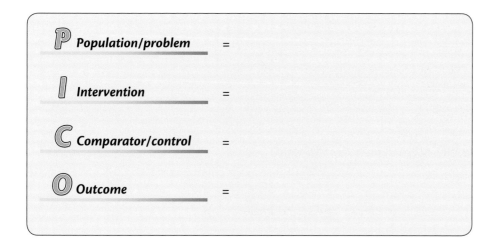

Question:

_____

_____

_____

Quiz: Formulate clinical questions

1. **Which of the following questions do you think is/are answerable by research?**
   a. What is the meaning of life?
   b. What is the risk of autism following a measles vaccine?
   c. What is the best treatment for osteoarthritis?
   d. Why don't patients take their prescribed medications?

2. **What is the implicit comparator in the following questions?**
   a. Does 'black cohosh' help with menopausal symptoms?
   b. Does high homocysteine mean a higher risk of cardiovascular disease?
   c. In otherwise well patients, does cloudy urine suggest a urinary tract infection?

3. **The following are the titles from a single issue of the BMJ. See if you can work out the PICO from the titles. Which parts are missing? What type of question is each and what study type has been used to answer it?**
   a. Effectiveness of discontinuing antibiotic treatment after three days versus eight days in mild to moderate–severe community-acquired pneumonia: randomised, double-blind study.
   b. Personality, lifestyle, and risk of cardiovascular disease and cancer: follow-up of population-based cohort.
   c. Colour of bile vomiting in intestinal obstruction in the newborn: questionnaire study.
   d. Effect of off-pump coronary artery bypass surgery on clinical, angiographic, neurocognitive, and quality-of-life outcomes: randomised controlled trial.

Answers to this quiz are in the 'Answers' section in Part 4 of this workbook.

Notes

EBP Step 2: Track down the best evidence

Steps in EBP

1. Formulate an answerable question.

2. Track down the best evidence of outcomes available.

3. Critically appraise the evidence (find out how good it is and what it means).

4. Apply the evidence (integrate the results with clinical expertise and patient values).

What study designs should you be looking for?

In EBP Step 1 (Formulate an answerable question), we saw that most clinical questions can be classified as being about interventions, aetiology and risk factors, diagnosis, prognosis, frequency and rate, or phenomena.

The types of studies that give the best evidence are different for the different types of questions. In every case, however, the best evidence comes from studies where the methods used maximise the chance of eliminating bias. (The issue of bias is discussed in detail in EBP Step 3: Critically appraise the studies.) The study designs that best suit the different question types are as follows:

Question	Best study designs*	Description
INTERVENTION	Randomised controlled trial (RCT)	Subjects are randomly allocated to treatment or control groups and outcomes assessed.
AETIOLOGY AND RISK FACTORS	Randomised controlled trial	As aetiology questions are similar to intervention questions, the ideal study type is an RCT. However, it is usually not ethical or practical to conduct such a trial to assess harmful outcomes.
	Cohort study	Outcomes are compared for matched groups with and without exposure or risk factor (prospective study).
	Case-control study	Subjects with and without outcome of interest are compared for previous exposure or risk factor (retrospective study).
FREQUENCY AND RATE	Cohort study	As above.
	Cross-sectional study	Measurement of condition in a representative (preferably random) sample of people.
DIAGNOSIS	Cross-sectional study with random or consecutive sample	Preferably an independent, blind, comparison with 'gold standard' test.
PROGNOSIS AND PREDICTION	Cohort /survival study	Long-term follow-up of a representative cohort.

* Descriptions of these study types are given in the 'Glossary' in Part 4 of this workbook. In each case, a systematic review of all the available studies is better than an individual study.

How to recognise different study types

These study designs all have similar components (as we'd expect from the PICO; see GATE graphic below):

- a defined population, from which groups of subjects are studied

- interventions or exposures that are applied to different groups of subjects

- outcomes that are measured.

Whether or not the researcher actively changes a factor or uses an intervention determines whether the study is considered to be observational (passive involvement of researcher) or experimental (active involvement of researcher).

Experimental studies are similar to experiments in other areas of science. That is, subjects are allocated to two or more groups to receive an intervention or exposure and then followed up under carefully controlled conditions. Such controlled trials, particularly if randomised and blinded, have the potential to control for most of the biases that can occur in scientific studies. However, whether this actually occurs depends on the quality of the study design and implementation, as we will see in the section of this workbook about critical appraisal (see EBP Step 3).

Observational studies investigate and record exposures (such as interventions or risk factors) and observe outcomes (such as disease) as they occur. Such studies may be purely descriptive or more analytical:

- Analytical studies include case-control studies, cohort studies and some population (cross-sectional) studies. These studies all include matched groups of subjects and assess associations between exposures and outcomes.

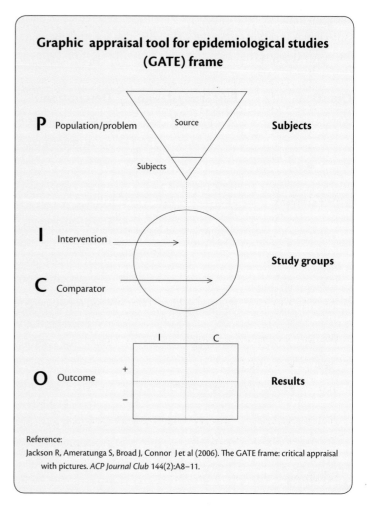

Graphic appraisal tool for epidemiological studies (GATE) frame

P Population/problem

I Intervention

C Comparator

O Outcome

Reference:
Jackson R, Ameratunga S, Broad J, Connor J et al (2006). The GATE frame: critical appraisal with pictures. *ACP Journal Club* 144(2):A8–11.

- Descriptive studies include case reports, case-series and some cross-sectional studies, which measure the frequency of several factors, and hence the size of the problem. They may sometimes also include analytic work (comparing factors).

The figure below shows the different types of studies arranged in a descending hierarchy from the least (top) to the most (bottom) biased. Brief descriptions of each study type are given in the 'Glossary' in Part 4 of this workbook.

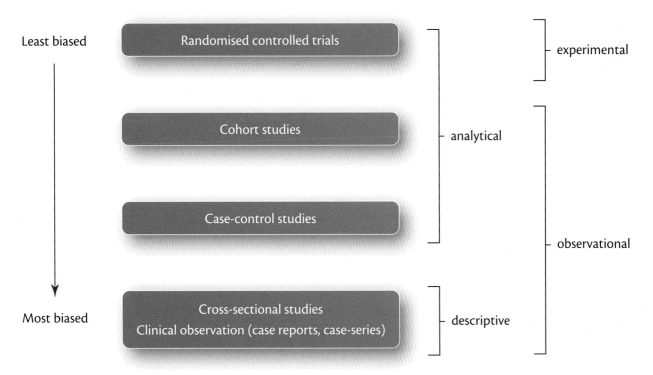

Hierarchy of study designs for interventions

The type of study can generally be worked out by looking at two issues:

1. **Was the intervention randomly allocated?**

    Yes ▶ RCT

    No ▶ Observational study

    The main types of observational study then depend on the timing of the measurement of outcome.

2. **When were the outcomes determined?**

    a. Some time after the exposure or intervention

        ▶ cohort study ('prospective study').

    b. At the same time as the exposure or intervention

        ▶ cross-sectional study or survey.

    c. Before the exposure was determined

        ▶ case-control study ('retrospective study' based on recall of the exposure).

The table below sets out a hierarchy of evidence that has been developed for each type of clinical question. Note that the table is a guide for searching, and only gives a rough initial assessment of the evidence, which may need to be adjusted after the quality of the study is assessed in detail (we will look at this in more detail in EBP Step 3 of this workbook).

Designation of levels of evidence according to type of research question

	Level	Intervention[1]	Diagnosis[2]	Prognosis[1]	Aetiology[1,3]
Least biased	I	Systematic review of level II studies	Systematic review of level II studies	Systematic review of level II studies	Systematic review of level II studies
	II	Randomised controlled trial	Cross-sectional study among consecutive presenting patients	Inception cohort study	Prospective cohort study
	III	One of the following: • non-randomised experimental study (eg controlled pre- and post-test intervention study) • comparative (observational) study with a concurrent control group (eg cohort study, case-control study)	One of the following: • cross-sectional study among non-consecutive patients • diagnostic case-control study	One of the following: • untreated control patients in a randomised controlled trial • retrospectively assembled cohort study	One of the following: • retrospective cohort study • case-control study (Note: these are the most common study types for aetiology, but see level III for intervention studies for other options)
Most biased	IV	Case series	Case series	Case series, or a cohort study of patients at different stages of disease	A cross-sectional study

1 In rare instances, 'all-or-none' evidence may be available for these types of questions (see Glossary) and, depending on the circumstances, may provide confirmation of effectiveness or causation.

2 These levels of evidence apply only to studies of diagnostic accuracy. To assess the *effectiveness* of a diagnostic test, there also needs to be a consideration of the impact of the test on patient management and health outcomes.

3 If it is possible and/or ethical to determine a causal relationship using *experimental* evidence, then the 'intervention' hierarchy of evidence can be used. If it is only possible and/or ethical to determine a causal relationship using observational evidence (eg because it is not possible to allocate groups to a potential harmful exposure, such as nuclear radiation), then this 'aetiology' hierarchy of evidence can be used.

Note: For definitions of the study designs, see the 'Glossary' in Part 4 of this workbook.

Source: Modified from the Centre for Evidence-Based Medicine (Oxford) website (http://www.cebm.net/levels_of_evidence.asp) and the National Health and Medical Research Council (Australia) (http://www.nhmrc.gov.au).

Exercise: Study designs

Read the following abstracts from published studies and answer the questions
that follow each study.

> **Abstract 1**

Voutilainen S, Rissanen TH, Virtanen J, Lakka TA, Salonen JT (2001). Low dietary folate intake
is associated with an excess incidence of acute coronary events: The Kuopio Ischemic Heart
Disease Risk Factor Study. *Circulation* 103(22):2674–2680.

Background: Although several prospective studies have shown that low folate intake and low
circulating folate are associated with increased risk of coronary heart disease (CHD), the findings
are inconsistent.

Methods and results: We studied the associations of dietary intake of folate, vitamin B6,
and vitamin B12 with the risk of acute coronary events in a prospective cohort study of 1980
Finnish men 42 to 60 years old, examined in 1984 to 1989 in the Kuopio Ischemic Heart
Disease Risk Factor Study. Nutrient intakes were assessed by 4-day food record. During an
average follow-up time of 10 years, 199 acute coronary events occurred. In a Cox proportional
hazards model adjusted for 21 conventional and nutritional CHD risk factors, men in the
highest fifth of folate intake had a relative risk of acute coronary events of 0.45 (95%CI 0.25
to 0.81, $P=0.008$) compared with men in the lowest fifth. This association was stronger in
non-smokers and light alcohol users than in smokers and alcohol users. A high dietary intake
of vitamin B6 had no significant association and that of vitamin B12 a weak association with a
reduced risk of acute coronary events.

Conclusions: The present work in CHD-free middle-aged men is the first prospective cohort
study to observe a significant inverse association between quantitatively assessed moderate-
to-high folate intakes and incidence of acute coronary events in men. Our findings provide
further support in favour of a role of folate in the promotion of good cardiovascular health.

Question	Answer
1. What is the question (PICO) of the study?	P
	I
	C
	O
2. What is the purpose of the study?	
3. Which primary study type would give the highest-quality evidence to answer the question?	
4. Which is the best study type that is also feasible?	
5. What is the study type used?	

Lonn E et al for the Heart Outcome Prevention Evaluation (HOPE) 2 Investigators (2006).
Homocysteine lowering with folic acid and B vitamins in vascular disease. *New England Journal of Medicine* 354(15):1567–1577.

Background: In observational studies, lower homocysteine levels are associated with lower rates of coronary heart disease and stroke. Folic acid and vitamins B6 and B12 lower homocysteine levels. We assessed whether supplementation reduced the risk of major cardiovascular events in patients with vascular disease.

Methods: We randomly assigned 5522 patients 55 years of age or older who had vascular disease or diabetes to daily treatment either with the combination of 2.5 mg of folic acid, 50 mg of vitamin B6 and 1 mg of vitamin B12, or with placebo for an average of five years. The primary outcome was a composite of death from cardiovascular causes, myocardial infarction and stroke.

Results: Mean plasma homocysteine levels decreased by 2.4 micromol per litre (0.3 mg per litre) in the active-treatment group and increased by 0.8 micromol per litre (0.1 mg per litre) in the placebo group. Primary outcome events occurred in 519 patients (18.8%) assigned to active therapy and 547 (19.8%) assigned to placebo (relative risk [RR] 0.95; 95% confidence interval [CI] 0.84 to 1.07; $P=0.41$). As compared with placebo, active treatment did not significantly decrease the risk of death from cardiovascular causes (relative risk 0.96; 95%CI 0.81 to 1.13), myocardial infarction (RR 0.98; 95%CI 0.85 to 1.14), or any of the secondary outcomes. Fewer patients assigned to active treatment than to placebo had a stroke (RR 0.75; 95%CI 0.59 to 0.97). More patients in the active-treatment group were hospitalized for unstable angina (RR 1.24; 95%CI 1.04 to 1.49).

Conclusions: Supplements combining folic acid and vitamins B6 and B12 did not reduce the risk of major cardiovascular events in patients with vascular disease.

Question	Answer
1. What is the question (PICO) of the study?	P
	I
	C
	O
2. What is the purpose of the study?	
3. Which primary study type would give the highest-quality evidence to answer the question?	
4. Which is the best study type that is also feasible?	
5. What is the study type used?	

Fitzpatrick MF, Martin K, Fossey E, Shapiro CM et al (1993). Snoring, asthma and sleep disturbance in Britain: a community-based survey. *European Respiratory Journal* 6(4):531–535.

A questionnaire was sent to a random sample of adults in eight locations throughout Britain, to investigate the prevalence of snoring, asthma and sleep complaints in community-based British adults. Of the 1478 respondents (831 females, 647 males; mean +/- SD age 45 +/- 18 years), 37% reported snoring at least occasionally, and 11% reported snoring on at least four nights per week (frequent snorers). Frequent snorers reported spending less time asleep at night, falling asleep accidentally during the day more often, taking planned daytime naps, and falling asleep whilst driving or operating machinery more often than the other respondents.

Using ordinal logistic regression analysis to allow for the age and sex of the respondents, both accidental daytime sleep and planned daytime naps were commoner in frequent snorers than other respondents. Six per cent of all respondents and 6% of those aged under 40 years reported that they had asthma (asthmatics). Seven per cent of respondents aged less than 40 years reported wheezing on three or more occasions per year, and had been prescribed oral or inhaled bronchodilators (young wheezers).

Question	Answer
1. What is the question (PICO) of the study?	P
	I
	C
	O
2. What is the purpose of the study?	
3. Which primary study type would give the highest-quality evidence to answer the question?	
4. Which is the best study type that is also feasible?	
5. What is the study type used?	

Chen SM, Chang MH, Du JC, Lin CC, Chen AC et al, Taiwan Infant Stool Color Card Study Group (2006). Screening for biliary atresia by infant stool color card in Taiwan. *Pediatrics* 117(4):1147-1154.

Objective: We aimed to detect biliary atresia (BA) in early infancy to prevent additional liver damage because of the delay of referral and surgical treatment and to investigate the incidence rate of BA in Taiwan.

Methods: A pilot study to screen the stool color in infants for the early diagnosis of BA was undertaken from March 2002 to December 2003. We had designed an 'infant stool color card' with 7 numbers of different color pictures and attached it to the child's health booklet. Parents were then asked to observe their infant's stool color by using this card. The medical staff would check the number that the parents chose according to their infant's stool color at 1 month of age during the health checkup and then send the card back to the stool color card registry center.

Results: The average return rate was approximately 65.2% (78,184 infants). A total of 29 infants were diagnosed as having BA, and 26 were screened out by stool color card before 60 days of age. The sensitivity, specificity, and positive predictive value were 89.7%, 99.9%, and 28.6%, respectively. Seventeen (58.6%) infants with BA received a Kasai operation within 60-day age period. The estimated incidence of BA in screened newborns was 3.7 of 10,000.

Conclusions: The stool color card was a simple, efficient, and applicable mass screening method for early diagnosis and management of BA. The program can also help in estimating the incidence and creating a registry of these patients.

Question	Answer
1. What is the question (PICO) of the study?	P
	I
	C
	O
2. What is the purpose of the study?	
3. Which primary study type would give the highest-quality evidence to answer the question?	
4. Which is the best study type that is also feasible?	
5. What is the study type used?	

Brna P, Dooley J, Gordon K, Dewan T (2005). The prognosis of childhood headache: a 20-year follow-up. *Archives of Pediatric and Adolescent Medicine* 159:1157-60.

Background: Headaches affect most children and rank third among illness-related causes of school absenteeism. Although the short-term outcome for most children appears favorable, few studies have reported long-term outcome.

Objective: To evaluate the long-term prognosis of childhood headaches 20 years after initial diagnosis in a cohort of Atlantic Canadian children who had headaches diagnosed in 1983.

Methods: Ninety-five patients with headaches who consulted 1 of the authors in 1983 were previously studied in 1993. The 77 patients contacted in 1993 were followed up in 2003. A standardized interview protocol was used.

Results: Sixty (78%) of 77 patients responded (60 of the 95 of the original cohort). At 20-year follow-up, 16 (27%) were headache free, 20 (33%) had tension-type headaches, 10 (17%) had migraine, and 14 (23%) had migraine and tension-type headaches. Having more than 1 headache type was more prevalent than at diagnosis or initial follow-up (P<.001), and headache type varied across time.

Conclusions: Twenty years after diagnosis of pediatric headache, most patients continue to have headache, although the headache classification often changes across time.

Question	Answer
1. What is the question (PICO) of the study?	P
	I
	C
	O
2. What is the purpose of the study?	
3. Which primary study type would give the highest-quality evidence to answer the question?	
4. Which is the best study type that is also feasible?	
5. What is the study type used?	

Answers to this abstract exercise are in the 'Answers' section in Part 4 of this workbook.

Organisation of evidence

The study types that we have been looking at above, such as RCTs, cohort studies or studies of diagnostic test accuracy, are all examples of 'primary research', whereas a systematic review is an example of 'secondary research' (that is, a collation of primary research to provide further insights into a topic).

In his article about the '4S' evolution of services for finding current best evidence, Brian Haynes describes four levels of organisation of evidence from research (see box).

In this representation, the primary research studies (RCTs, cohort studies, diagnostic accuracy studies, etc) are at the base of the triangle. Above these are three levels of secondary research (ie collations of evidence from primary studies) in ascending order of usefulness to busy practitioners. Unfortunately, the top level, which Haynes called 'systems', is not yet very well developed, although there are some attempts to move the organisation of clinical evidence in this direction.

There are some useful examples of the next level (ie synopses), however, such as the ACP Journal Club, the *Evidence-Based Medicine* series of journals and the BMJ's *Clinical Evidence*. Further information and examples of these synopses are in Part 4 of this workbook. These are useful sources of information for busy practitioners, because the task of reading and assimilating primary and more detailed secondary research has already been done, and the conclusion is presented in an easy-to-use form to support clinical decision making. Other examples of syntheses that are used for clinical decision making are clinical practice guidelines and decision aids.

Below these synopses are the more detailed accounts of secondary research, such as the systematic reviews found in The Cochrane Library. Haynes called these 'syntheses'.

In this section of the workbook, we will focus on the quickest ways of finding the most relevant primary studies, secondary studies (syntheses) and, where applicable, synopses to answer your clinical questions.

'4S' evolution of services

Examples

Systems — Computerised decision support systems (CDSS)

Synopses — Evidence-based journal abstracts

Syntheses — Cochrane reviews

Studies — Original published articles in journals

Reference:

Haynes RB (2001). Of studies, syntheses, synopses and systems: the '4S' evolution of services for finding best evidence. *Evidence-Based Medicine* 6:36–38. (The full article is included in the 'Further reading' section in Part 4 of this workbook.)

Where to search

PubMed

National Library of Medicine free internet MEDLINE database, with more than 10 million research entries dating back to 1966.

http://www.pubmed.gov

The 'Clinical Queries' section of PubMed is a question-focused interface with filters for identifying the more appropriate studies for questions of therapy, prognosis, diagnosis and aetiology. You will find this in the middle of the PubMed Services list on the left hand side of the main PubMed page.

The Cochrane Library

The Cochrane Library is mainly concerned with intervention studies. It contains all the reviews, trials, and other information collected by The Cochrane Collaboration. It contains the following databases:

The Cochrane Database of Systematic Reviews	Cochrane systematic reviews, with more than 2000 systematic reviews across all medical topics.
The Database of Abstracts of Reviews of Effectiveness (DARE)	Structured abstracts of systematic reviews.
The Cochrane Controlled Trials Register (CENTRAL)	Register of clinical trials that have been carried out or are in progress. The register contains more than 400,000 controlled trials, which is the best single repository in the world.

Access to the Cochrane Library is free for all users in the United Kingdom, Australia, and several other countries.

Go to **http://www.cochrane.org** and follow the prompts

Clinical Evidence

The BMJ's publication, *Clinical Evidence*, is a directory of evidence on the effects of clinical interventions. It summarises the current state of knowledge, ignorance and uncertainty about the prevention and treatment of clinical conditions, based on thorough searches and appraisal of the literature (particularly Cochrane reviews). *Clinical Evidence* covers about 30 speciality areas and includes more than 200 medical conditions. It is updated every six months and is available in print, on CD and online (by subscription).

See: **http://www.clinicalevidence.com**

Other useful places to search

Elsevier publish a subscription-only database called EMBASE, which contains a number of citations not in MEDLINE, especially in areas relating to drug development and use.

See: **http://www.embase.com**

Further useful sources are listed in 'Useful sources of evidence' in Part 4 of this workbook.

The question guides the search

In the previous section, we discussed how to break down any type of clinical question into four components:

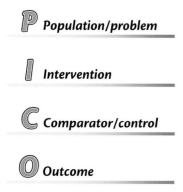

P *Population/problem*

I *Intervention*

C *Comparator/control*

O *Outcome*

You can now use these components to direct your search.

General structure of question

> (Population OR synonym1 OR synonym2...) AND
>
> (Intervention OR synonym1 OR synonym2...) AND
>
> (Comparator OR synonym1 OR synonym2...) AND
>
> (Outcome OR synonym1 OR synonym2...)

Example:

Question: In adults screened with faecal occult blood testing, compared with no screening, is there a reduction in the mortality from colorectal cancer?

Question part	Question term	Synonyms
Population/problem	Adult, human, colorectal cancer	Bowel cancer, colorectal neoplasm
Intervention	Screening	Screen, early detection
Comparator	No screening	–
Outcome	Mortality	Death, survival

In looking for synonyms, you should consider both textwords and keywords in the database you are searching. The MEDLINE keyword system, which is known as MeSH (Medical Subject Heading), has a tree structure that covers a broad set of synonyms very quickly. The 'explode' (exp) feature of the tree structure allows you to capture an entire subtree of MeSH terms within a single word. Thus for the colorectal cancer term in the above search, the appropriate MeSH term might be:

```
colonic neoplasm (exp)
```

with the 'explode' incorporating all the MeSH tree below colonic neoplasm, as follows:

```
colorectal neoplasms
        colonic polyps
                adenomatous polyposis coli
        colorectal neoplasms
                colorectal neoplasms, hereditary
                nonpolyposis
        sigmoid neoplasms
```

While the MeSH system is useful, it should supplement rather than usurp the use of textwords so that incompletely coded articles are not missed. The MeSH site can be accessed from PubMed (see 'How to use PubMed' later in this section).

The parts of the question can also be represented as a Venn diagram:

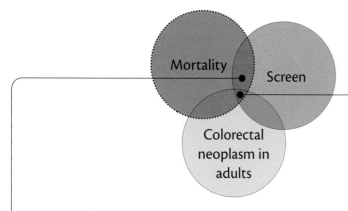

Once the study question has been broken down into its components, they can be combined using the Boolean operators 'AND' and 'OR'. For example:

➤ `(mortality AND screen)` — represents the overlap between these two terms — retrieves only articles that use both terms.

`(screen AND colorectal neoplasm AND mortality)` ◄ — represents the small area where all three circles overlap — retrieves only articles with all three terms.

Complex combinations are possible. For example, the following combination captures all the overlap areas between the circles in the Venn diagram:

`(mortality AND screen) OR (mortality AND colorectal neoplasms) OR (screen AND colorectal neoplasms)`

Although the overlap of all the parts of the question will generally have the best concentration of relevant articles, the other areas may still contain many relevant articles. Hence, if the disease AND study factor combination (solid circles in Venn diagram) is manageable, it is best to work with this and not further restrict by, for example, using outcomes (dotted circle in Venn diagram above).

When the general structure of the question is developed it is worth looking for synonyms for each component.

Thus a full PICO search might be:

`(screen* OR early detection) AND (colorectal cancer OR bowel cancer) AND (mortality OR death* OR survival)`

The term 'screen*' is shorthand for words beginning with screen, for example, screen, screened, screening. (Note: the 'wildcard' symbol varies between systems, eg it may be an asterisk [*], or colon [:].)

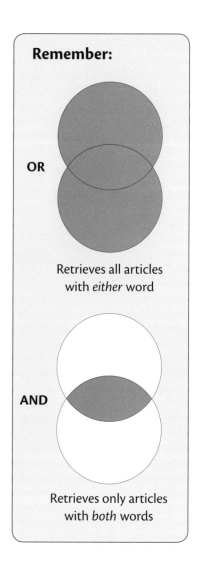

Remember:

OR

Retrieves all articles with *either* word

AND

Retrieves only articles with *both* words

Searching tips and tactics

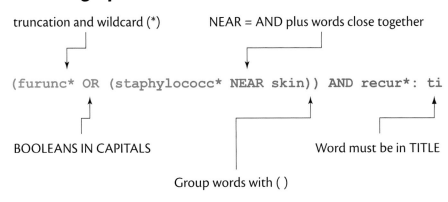

truncation and wildcard (*)   NEAR = AND plus words close together

`(furunc* OR (staphylococc* NEAR skin)) AND recur*: ti`

BOOLEANS IN CAPITALS   Word must be in TITLE

Group words with ( )

PubMed command	What it does	Some synonyms (eg OVID)
OR	Finds studies containing either of the specified words or phrases. For example, `child OR adolescent` finds articles with either the word 'child' or the word 'adolescent'.	
AND	Finds studies containing both specified words or phrases. For example, `child AND adolescent` finds articles with both the word 'child' and the word 'adolescent'.	+
NEAR	Like **AND**, **NEAR** requires both words but the specified words must also be within about 5 words of each other. It is not available in PubMed but is in other MEDLINE interfaces.	ADJ
NOT	Excludes studies containing the specified word or phrase. For example, `child NOT adolescent` means studies with the word 'child' but not the word 'adolescent'. Use sparingly.	−
Limits	Articles retrieved may be restricted in several ways. For example, by date, by language, by whether there is an abstract, etc.	
()	Use parentheses to group words. For example, `(child OR adolescent) AND (hearing OR auditory)` finds articles with one or both 'child' and 'adolescent' and one or both of the words 'hearing' or 'auditory'.	
*	Truncation: the '*' acts as a wildcard indicating any further letters. For example, child* is child plus any further letters and is equivalent to `(child OR childs OR children OR childhood)`. Note that wildcards turn off automatic MeSH mapping in PubMed.	$
[ti] or:ti	Finds studies with the word in the title. For example, `hearing[ti]` finds studies with the word hearing in the title.	:ti (Cochrane)
so or [so]	Retrieves studies from a specific source. For example, `hearing AND BMJ[so]` finds articles on hearing in the BMJ.	
MeSH	MeSH is the Medical Subject Headings, a controlled vocabulary of keywords that may be used in PubMed or Cochrane. It is often useful to use both MeSH heading and text words (see section on 'How to use PubMed', below).	
" "	Use of quote marks will ask the database to search the phrase dictionary for that phrase. If none is found the words are simply joined by AND.	

Computer searching

Our workshop computers will be set to use PubMed and The Cochrane Library. What to search for depends on the type of question you have asked. For an intervention question, the best evidence comes from a systematic review of RCTs, and the best systematic reviews are in The Cochrane Database of Systematic Reviews in The Cochrane Library. Ideally, you should start searching at the level that will give you the best possible evidence (see the table of levels of evidence on page 42). If you do not find anything, drop down to the next level.

However, most Cochrane reviews are also indexed in PubMed so we recommend that, even for intervention questions, you start your search by looking at PubMed Clinical Queries. Then, if you have time, or want to follow up more thoroughly later on, you can do a more thorough search of The Cochrane Library, including the DARE database (a DARE review is the next best evidence after a Cochrane review, so if there is one, you do not need to look further). The Clinical Trials Register will also tell you if any trials are in progress.

The search path you can follow to find **studies** and **syntheses** for most questions is shown in the flowchart on the following page.

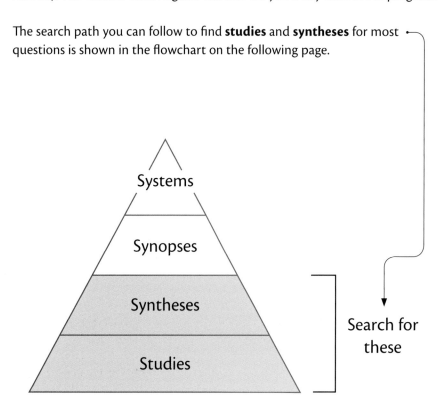

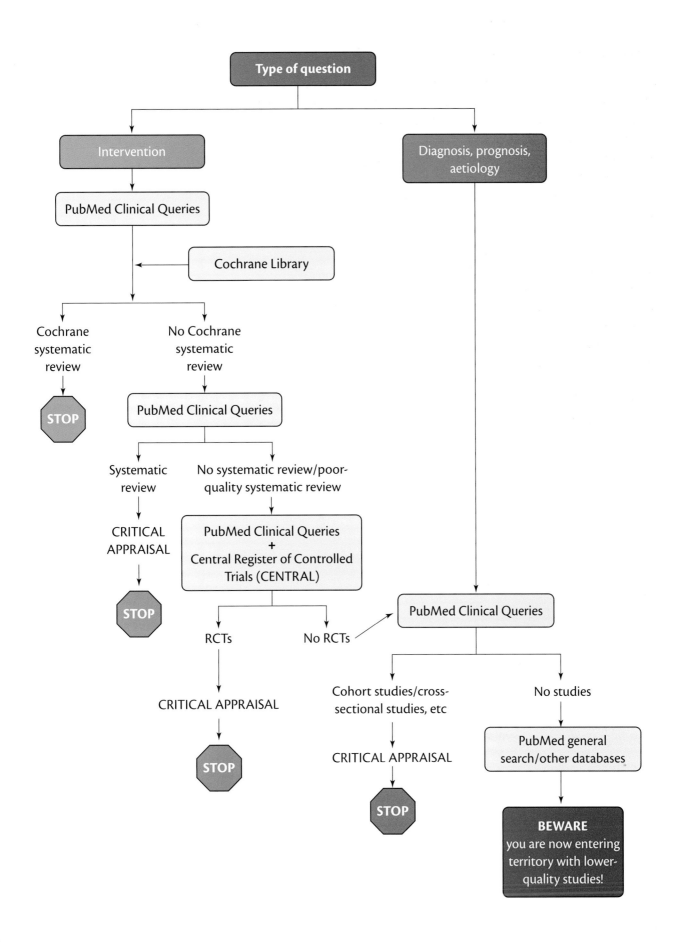

How to use PubMed

Go to the 'Entrez-PubMed' webpage at:

http://www.ncbi.nlm.nih.gov/entrez/query.fcgi

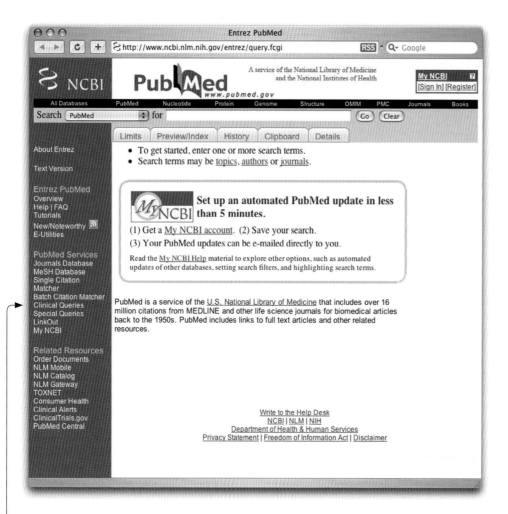

You can search directly from the entry page by typing your search terms into the box at the top. Click 'Limits' to set limits such as date, language and type of article. However, this sort of search does not provide any filtering for quality of the research and you will probably retrieve a large number of articles of variable usefulness.

To improve the quality of the studies you retrieve, click on 'Clinical Queries' on the sidebar.

The screenshots on pages 56–58 are reproduced with permission. Source: The National Center for Biotechnology Information, The National Library of Medicine, The National Institute of Health, Department of Health and Human Services.

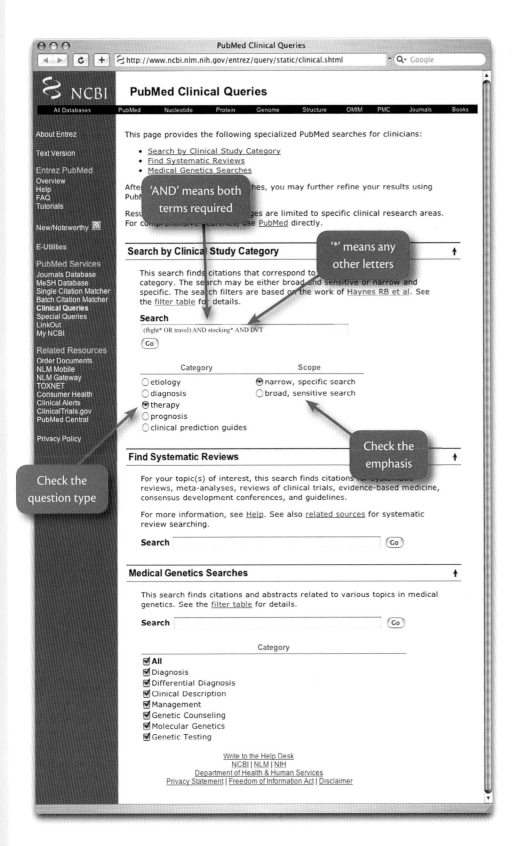

Next, enter the type of question you are trying to answer (ie intervention [therapy], diagnosis, aetiology, prognosis). If you click the 'Sensitivity' button you will get more articles but some may be less relevant. 'Specificity' gives you only highly relevant articles.

Finally, enter your search terms in the box and click 'Go'.

More about MeSH headings

From the PubMed entry page, click 'MeSH Browser' from the sidebar. In the next screen click 'MeSH'.

Next, click 'Online searching' to enter the search browser. Now you can enter the term you are looking for to get the full MeSH subject heading list for that topic.

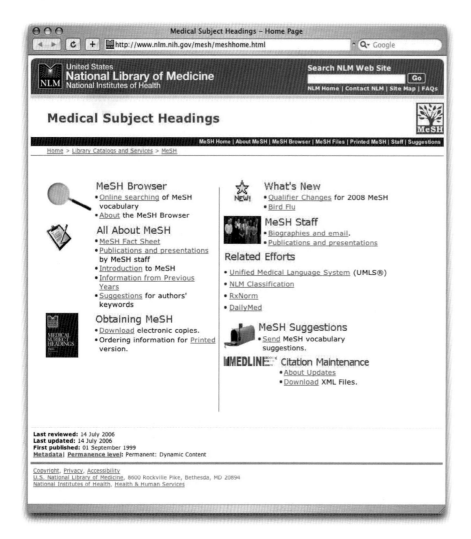

PubMed tutorial

PubMed has a detailed tutorial program. Click on 'Tutorial' on the side bar of the PubMed entry page. The tutorial is quite detailed and takes about two hours to go right through, but it is very helpful.

How to use The Cochrane Library

Go to The Cochrane Library by following the prompts from:
http://www.cochrane.org

If you are in a registered country for use of the library, you will automatically be able to log on to use the library.

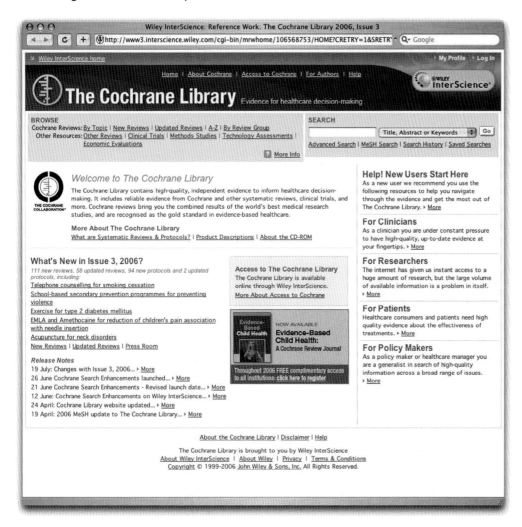

As noted on page 49, the library includes:

- the Cochrane Database of Systematic Reviews

- the Database of Abstracts of Reviews of Effectiveness

- The Cochrane Controlled Trials Register (CENTRAL), which lists more than 300,000 controlled trials that have been carried out or are currently in progress

- some other databases (methods, etc).

Screenshot from John Wiley & Sons, Inc.'s World Wide Website.
© 1999-2007 John Wiley & Sons, Inc. Reprinted with permission.

To search the library, enter your search phrase in the space provided. The results will show the total 'hits' from the site and the hits from each database. Click on each report to show the details.

Cochrane systematic reviews are very detailed but each has a structured abstract with the main findings. You can also go to the 'Graphs' section towards the end of the report and click on the studies to see the results of the analysis. These results can often be used to calculate a 'number needed to treat' (NNT).

For example, the search terms 'carpal tunnel AND corticosteroid' shows the following systematic review:

'Local corticosteroid treatment for carpal tunnel syndrome'

The 'Graphs' section of the review shows one study where corticosteroid treatment was compared to placebo treatment with the numbers of patients showing improvement at 1 month as the outcome.

The results showed a statistically significant benefit at one month for the treated group of patients as follows:

	Number improved at 1 month	% improved
Hydrocortisone	23/30	77
Placebo	6/30	20
Percentage improved because of treatment		57 (57 better from 100 treated)
NNT		100/57 = 1.75 (ie more than 1 in every 2 patients treated will improve)

Note: Symptom improvement beyond 1 month has not been demonstrated.

Searching 'warm-up'

Before you start to search for a study to answer the question you formulated in the earlier section, we will walk through the search process with an example question.

Step 1: Create a search strategy

Scenario: A 64-year-old obese male who has tried many ways to lose weight presents with a newspaper article about 'fat-blazer' (chitosan). He asks for your advice.

Your question in PICO format might be:

P **Population/problem** = obese patients

I **Intervention** = chitosan

C **Comparator/control** = placebo

O **Outcome** = decreased weight

Question: In obsese patients, does chitosan, compared with a placebo, decrease weight?

Step 2: Convert this question to a search strategy

To do this, first do 3 things:

1. Underline the key terms.

2. Number in order of importance from 1 to 4.

3. Think of alternative spellings, synonyms and truncations.

You might end up with:

P *Population/problem*   =   obes* OR overweight (2)

I *Intervention*   =   chitosan (1)

C *Comparator/control*   =   placebo (4)

O *Outcome*   =   decrease weight OR kilogram* (3)

NOTE:

'*' is a truncation symbol that means further letters can be added to the word.

OR finds studies containing either of the specified words/phrases, and broadens your search.

AND finds studies containing both specified words/phrases, and narrows your search.

Next, run through the following exercise:

1. Open your browser (eg Explorer) and go to http://www.pubmed.gov

2. Type in the term we chose as (1): 'chitosan'. Write down the number of results you found....

3. Select Clinical Queries (left-hand menu)

4. Select the Therapy category (which is the default) and search on 'chitosan' again. Write down the number of results you now found ....

Why has this decreased? It is because of the 'filter' that PubMed uses to focus on clinical trials (to see the actual filter click on the 'filter table' on the Clinical Queries page).

5. Try adding 'AND another stage', ie type in chitosan AND (obes* OR overweight) — note that you need brackets around your OR search. This should reduce the number of articles even further and certainly down to a manageable number.

If we had used all terms, the search may have looked like this:

Search #1:   chitosan
Search #2:   obes* OR overweight
Search #3:   weight OR kilogram*
Search #4:   placebo
Search #5:   #1 AND #2 AND #3 AND #4

However, you might have found that the first 1 or 2 search terms were enough to narrow down the search to around 20 titles.

Now apply the search strategy to a database, using the Search History button to view and combine the stages of your search.

Your own questions

Now return to the clinical questions that you developed in EBP Step 1 (Formulate an answerable question).

Use the table below to write down some search terms that you can use to get going on the search, based on your PICO and synonyms. Number the terms in order of importance:

Question 1:		
Question part	**Question term**	**Synonyms**
P Population/problem	(OR	)AND
I Intervention	(OR	)AND
C Comparator/control	(OR	)AND
O Outcome	(OR	)
Results of search		

Remember to consider truncating words and using the * wildcard symbol, for example: child* rather than children.

Question 2:		
Question part	**Question term**	**Synonyms**
P *Population/problem*	(	OR	)AND
I *Intervention*	(	OR	)AND
C *Comparator/control*	(	OR	)AND
O *Outcome*	(	OR	)

For intervention questions, you should try searching both PubMed and The Cochrane Library.

We suggest the following steps for PubMed Clinical Queries:

1. Go to http://www.pubmed.gov and select Clinical Queries (left-hand menu).

2. Select the appropriate category (usually 'therapy', which is the default).

3. Type in the most crucial element of your PICO search (usually the I or the P).

4. If your search returns no articles then click the 'Broad' scope.

5. If your search returns more than 30 articles then try adding more terms. For example, if you used only the 'I' now try searching the I AND P (use capitals for the AND).

6. Select the best single article (eg the largest or longest trial NOT necessarily the most recent). Please record why you chose the article you did.

Use the 'Results' tables on the next two pages for each of the questions to record the different words/phrases you used, the number of hits, and the final 'best evidence' you chose.

Results

Question 1:

Cochrane Library search terms used:	Hits
Key references:	
Results (including absolute risk, NNT, etc if possible):	
PubMed search terms used:	Hits
Key references:	
Results (including absolute risk, NNT, etc if possible):	

Question 2:

Cochrane Library search terms used:	Hits

Key references:

Results (including absolute risk, NNT, etc if possible):

PubMed search terms used:	Hits

Key references:

Results (including absolute risk, NNT, etc if possible):

Reporting back

Report back on what you found out during your literature searching session. Discuss WHAT you found and HOW you found it. Try to include empirical evidence, such as the NNT.

Literature search findings:

Quiz: Track down the best evidence

1. Which study type is best?

For the issues described below (examples 1 to 4), choose the SINGLE most relevant study type from those listed (options A to F) and write the letter of your chosen option in the space provided at the end of the example:

The best type of study to assess:

1. the effect of a new *treatment* would be _____
2. the *prevalence* of cataracts would be _____
3. the accuracy of a new *diagnostic test* would be _____
4. the *natural history (prognosis)* would be _____

Options:

A. a cohort study

B. a case-control study

C. a randomised controlled trial

D. a population survey

E. a consecutive sample of patients with a reference standard test

F. a qualitative study

2. Choose the SINGLE most relevant term from those listed (options A to L) to fill in the blanks for the search issues listed:

1. keywords coded by the National Library of Medicine are _____
2. requires that an article contains BOTH words _____
3. is used to find words with the same stem _____
4. contains the largest database of randomised controlled trials _____
5. requires that an article contains EITHER word _____
6. is a MEDLINE interface available free via the internet _____
7. to use all subheadings of a MESH term you would use an _____
8. contains the largest database of non-randomised studies _____

Options:

A. MeSH terms   E. OR   I. OVID

B. limiters   F. NOT   J. The Cochrane Library

C. PubMed   G. wildcard (*)   K. MEDLINE

D. AND   H. EMBASE   L. explode

3. Read the examples below (A, B). For each, indicate whether they are formulated to correctly search for an answer to the question (tick either YES or NO where indicated).

Example A: What strategies can be used to minimise falls in our elderly population?

Search: elderly or (old and prevent* and fall) or fracture

Is this search correctly formulated?   ☐ Yes   ☐ No

If no, what is the correct formulation?   _____

_____

Example B: Does ginkgo biloba raise blood pressure (or cause hypertension)?

Search: ginkgo OR blood OR pressure OR hypertension

Is this search correctly formulated?   ☐ Yes   ☐ No

If no, what is the correct formulation?   _____

_____

Answers to this quiz are in the 'Answers' section in Part 4 of this workbook.

Notes

EBP Step 3: Critically appraise the evidence

In the previous sections, you found out how to formulate clinical questions, how to identify the best types of evidence for different study types, and how to search for the best studies. The next step is to have a careful look at the study or studies you found and decide how good they are for answering your clinical question. This process is called '**critical appraisal**'.

We saw in EBP Step 2 (Track down the best evidence) that, for each type of clinical question, there is a hierarchy of evidence. The study types most likely to give the best evidence are at the top of the hierarchy with other, less reliable, study types in order below it. In each case, the likely best evidence (level I) is a systematic review of several of the best individual studies (level II) – provided the review is up to date and well done!

In EBP Step 2, we also saw that if your clinical question is an intervention question and you are lucky enough to find a Cochrane systematic review, you will not have to think much further about the quality of the individual studies included in the review. This is because Cochrane reviewers follow a rigorous protocol of critical appraisal, and you can *usually* be assured that the included studies are valid and the conclusions drawn are accurate, based on the data available – but you should at least check the search date of the review to see if it is up to date.

But what if you did not find a Cochrane review and instead found either one or a few individual studies or other types of reviews? This section will teach you the key quality features to look for in individual studies (**primary research**) and reviews (**secondary research**) to quickly determine whether the results are valid and clinically useful.

The section is illustrated by practice exercises and worked examples from the medical literature for critical appraisal of a primary research study (a randomised controlled trial, or RCT) and a secondary research study (a systematic review) to answer an intervention question.

Part 3 of this workbook provides examples, brief notes and worksheets to show how these same principles can be applied to the appraisal of studies that answer different clinical questions (prognosis and diagnosis).

The aim of all the exercises in this section and in Part 3 is to help you critically appraise a variety of study types consistently, reliably and — most importantly — rapidly!

Steps in EBP

1. Formulate an answerable question.

2. Track down the best evidence of outcomes available.

3. Critically appraise the evidence (find out how good it is and what it means).

4. Apply the evidence (integrate the results with clinical expertise and patient values).

Principles of critical appraisal — primary research

Primary research in health care is about measuring differences between groups of subjects who undergo different clinical interventions, or are exposed to different risk factors, or have different characteristics, etc. As for research on other complex biological systems, there are many things that can go wrong, depending on how well the studies are designed and executed.

Just because a study is the 'best' type of study (by the study hierarchy) for our clinical question (such as an RCT for an intervention question), we can't necessarily be confident of the study's conclusions. Studies can be done very well or very badly (or anything in between). Thus, the type of study (level of evidence) is only a first dimension of the evidence that affects the confidence we can ultimately have in the authors' conclusions. The other dimensions can be determined using critical appraisal.

Critical appraisal of primary research involves three overall questions:

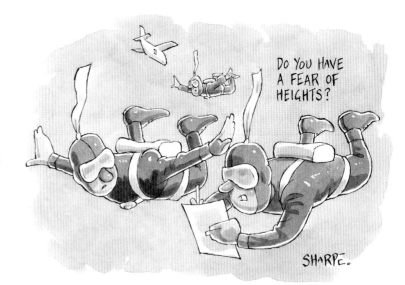

▶ Question 1: What is the PICO of the study, and is it close enough to your PICO?

▶ Question 2: How well was the study done?

▶ Question 3: What do the results mean and could they have been due to chance?

In this section, we will consider the principles involved in answering these questions and apply these principles to an RCT of the use of elastic stockings to reduce the risk of deep vein thrombosis (DVT) on long-haul airplane flights. See shaded sections with the logo: ✈

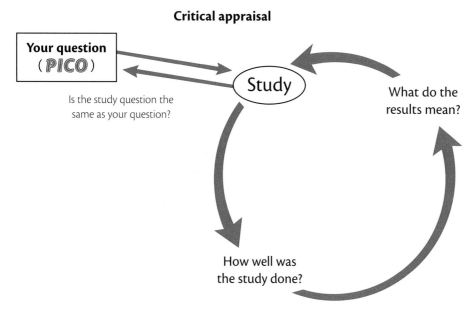

72

Critical appraisal of an intervention study

To illustrate the principles of critical appraisal for primary research, we will consider a topical intervention question for air travellers —whether wearing elastic stockings on long-haul flights helps to prevent deep vein thrombosis (DVT). Imagine that our PICO was as follows:

P *Population/problem* = passengers on long-haul flights

I *Intervention* = wearing elastic compression stockings

C *Comparator/control* = no elastic stockings

O *Outcome* = symptomless DVT

Clinical question

In passengers on long-haul flights, does wearing elastic compression stockings, compared to not wearing elastic stockings, prevent DVT?

Search terms

Based on the clinical question (PICO), we used the following search terms:

(flight* OR travel*) AND stocking* AND (DVT OR thrombosis)

Search results

PubMed Clinical Queries (therapy, broad), 20 hits (referring to 5 studies and several reviews, including one recent Cochrane review)

For this exercise we have chosen the following study to look at in more detail:

Scurr et al (2001). Frequency and prevention of symptomless deep-vein thrombosis in long-haul flights: a randomised trial. *The Lancet* 357:1485–1489.

Authors' conclusion

'Wearing of elastic compression stockings during long-haul air travel is associated with a reduction in symptomless DVT.'

The full paper is included on pages 95–99 of this workbook.

But how do we know that the results are valid and real? Wearing elastic stockings is an intervention so we know that the best type of primary research is an RCT (level II), and the study by Scurr et al is, indeed, an RCT but how confident can we be in this conclusion? In the following pages we will use the principles of critical appraisal to find out.

Note: This search revealed several primary studies and a number of review articles. In 'real life' you would go straight to the Cochrane systematic review — and check if it post-dated the individual trials — as this would provide the best evidence. If there was no systematic review, you would need to critically appraise the largest (and sometimes several) of the individual studies. However, for the purpose of this exercise, we have selected the slightly older study because it is shorter and easier to follow than the other two.

Question 1: Is the PICO of the study close enough to your PICO?

When you find a study that you think will help to answer your clinical question, the first thing to look at is whether the PICO of the study matches the PICO of your question. This helps to orient you to the paper and allows you to decide if it really provides useful information relevant to your PICO.

The study will rarely *exactly* match your question, so you will need to judge whether it is a close enough match to assist with your clinical decision. For example, your PICO may be:

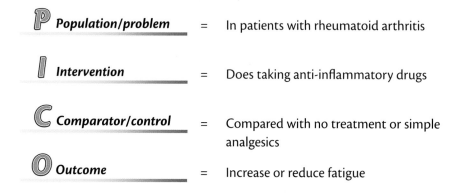

P *Population/problem*	=	In patients with rheumatoid arthritis
I *Intervention*	=	Does taking anti-inflammatory drugs
C *Comparator/control*	=	Compared with no treatment or simple analgesics
O *Outcome*	=	Increase or reduce fatigue

But the paper you have found may be about whether taking anti-inflammatory drugs reduces joint pain. That is, the 'PIC' are the same as yours but the 'O' is joint pain rather than fatigue. However, the study may have reported on some measures of fatigue (which patients often consider as the most important symptom) as a secondary outcome; or it may contain other information that is useful for your question. Therefore, the first step is to quickly decide if you want to appraise it further or not.

Other important differences between your PICO and the study PICO may be, for example, if your question is about children and the study population is adults; or if your question is about elderly people (over 70 years, for example) and the study population is middle-aged people. In such situations, you may have to think very carefully about whether the study is useful to answer your question. We will discuss this issue in more detail at EBP Step 4 (Apply the evidence).

Is the PICO of the DVT study close enough to your PICO?

Looking at the DVT trial, the PICO can be identified from the Summary section. It is much the same as our PICO, although the population is limited to people over 50 years of age. You would probably accept this as similar enough to be relevant. If the PICO of the study is significantly different from your clinical question, you may decide not to bother with the appraisal and continue your searching. However, in this case, it looks as though it is worth continuing.

Question 2: How well was the study done?

The quality of an epidemiological study — which is also referred to as its internal validity — is based on how well the research methods prevented the results from being affected by bias and confounding factors.

Bias is the degree to which the result is skewed away from the truth. It often reflects the human tendency to either consciously or subconsciously 'help' things work out the way we think they should. For researchers, this may be towards the results they want to support their theories. For subjects, it might be to suit their preconceptions of what should be happening to them (such as getting better when they take a pill). Bias is different from random error, or scatter, which occurs because of various system variables and is evenly distributed around the true mean.

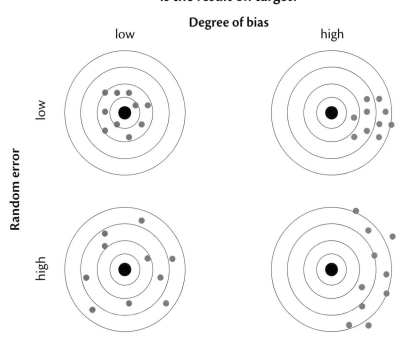

Is the result on target?

Unfortunately, bias seems to come in many shapes and sizes — bias in the way subjects are selected for a study, bias in the way they are allocated to groups, bias in the way groups are treated, bias in the way that measurements are made — to name but a few!

The best way to overcome this bias is to use study designs that keep as many people in the dark as possible about which intervention is which and remove the need for researcher and subject involvement in the process as much as possible. This includes selection of the subjects for the study, allocation to groups and measurement of outcomes.

Confounding factors are patient features and other possible causal factors, apart from the one that is being measured, that can affect the outcome of the study. To eliminate confounding factors, we need to ensure that the groups are as closely matched as possible at the start of the study and that management of the groups is the same in every respect apart from the treatment or exposure of interest.

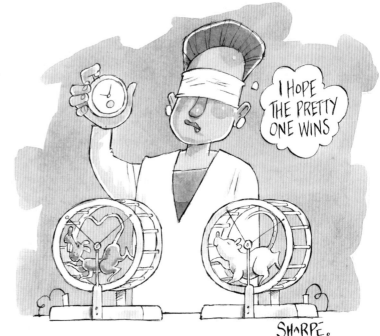

To find out how well bias and confounding factors were avoided in a health care study, you need to check each stage of the study to see how well bias has been eliminated or, to put it another way, how 'fairly' the study has been done; that is:

▶   How fairly were the subjects recruited (the 'P')?

▶   How fairly were the subjects allocated to groups (the 'I' and 'C')?

▶   How fairly were the study groups maintained through equal management and follow-up of subjects (the 'I' and 'C')?

▶   How fairly were the outcomes measured (the 'O')?

If the study that you have identified has eliminated bias, then there is a good chance that the study's results (which answer the PICO) will be reliable ... But how can you tell? The following sections describe the main factors to look out for.

In the figure opposite, we have related these questions to study methods that are most likely to eliminate bias (ie are fairest). These elements form the acronym '**RAMMbo**'. Each RAMMbo element is discussed below. The shaded boxes illustrate how these elements apply to an RCT, using the DVT trial as an example.

Structure of a comparative health care research study (primary research)

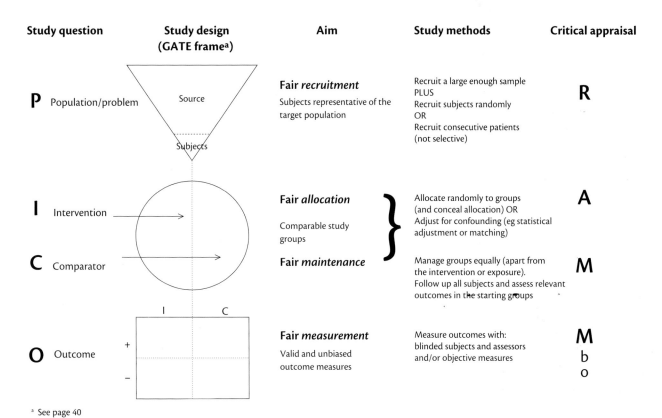

Study question	Study design (GATE frame[a])	Aim	Study methods	Critical appraisal
P Population/problem	Source · Subjects	**Fair *recruitment*** Subjects representative of the target population	Recruit a large enough sample PLUS Recruit subjects randomly OR Recruit consecutive patients (not selective)	**R**
I Intervention		**Fair *allocation*** Comparable study groups	Allocate randomly to groups (and conceal allocation) OR Adjust for confounding (eg statistical adjustment or matching)	**A**
C Comparator		**Fair *maintenance***	Manage groups equally (apart from the intervention or exposure). Follow up all subjects and assess relevant outcomes in the starting groups	**M**
O Outcome		**Fair *measurement*** Valid and unbiased outcome measures	Measure outcomes with: blinded subjects and assessors and/or objective measures	**M** **b** **o**

a See page 40

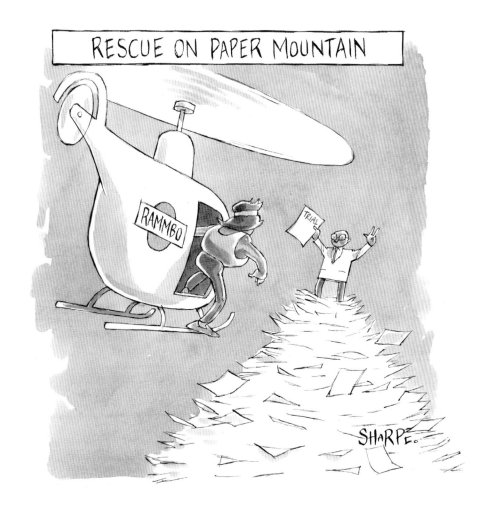

RESCUE ON PAPER MOUNTAIN

Recruitment — Were the subjects representative of the target population?

It is important that the subjects selected for a study appropriately represent the population of interest (the source population; for example, men, adults, women over 50 years). If the subjects of the study are not representative of a definable source population (e.g. a particular risk group or etiologic group), then it may be difficult to know to which population(s) the outcomes may be applicable — we can't be sure one way or the other.

The best way to ensure that the study groups are representative is to:

▶ recruit potential subjects sequentially (or at random from the whole population of interest) and clearly describe the source of patients; for example, first presentation or emergency presentation)

▶ only apply exclusion criteria that are relevant for the study methods (such as excluding deaf people from a study requiring subjects to listen to music) and not those that are based on other characteristics (such as weight or height in the case of a hearing study).

Other things being equal, we also prefer 'large' studies because small study groups provide an imprecise estimate of the effects. However, the number of subjects required for a meaningful study varies with the type of outcome studied. For continuous outcomes (such as height or weight), 50–100 might be sufficient. For events (or binary outcomes), such as a heart attack, the number of subjects required depends on how common the event of interest is. For common events, a trial may only require hundreds of subjects whereas rare events will only be captured with thousands of subjects.

There are also some 'rule-of-thumb' principles for working out how many subjects are needed in a specific study. These principles (dubbed 'cafe rules' because they can be used over a cup of coffee) are described in the paper by Glasziou and Doll 'Was the study big enough? Two cafe rules', which is included in the 'Further reading' section in Part 4 of this workbook. The first rule is that we need around 50 'events' in the control group; for example, if the expected event rate is 10% we need 500 people in each arm. The statistical application of these principles is also discussed below in the section on what the results show.

Steps in critical appraisal of primary research

Recruitment

Were the subjects representative of the target population?

Allocation or adjustment

Was the treatment allocation concealed before randomisation and were the groups comparable at the start of the trial?

Maintenance

Was the comparable status of the study groups maintained through equal management and adequate follow-up?

Measurement

Were the outcomes measured with:

blinded subjects and assessors, and/or

objective outcomes?

Recruitment — Were the DVT trial subjects representative of the target population?

Inclusion/exclusion criteria

For experimental studies, including RCTs, it is difficult to obtain a sequential or random sample of the population to be tested because of the need for consent. This means that such studies generally will not be representative of the whole population with a specific problem, so we need a clear idea of who they do represent. Therefore, the study should clearly describe the severity, duration and/or risk level of the patients recruited to ensure that the target population is adequately defined (this is the 'P', or population/problem, of the study).

Recruitment in the DVT trial was on a volunteer basis and volunteers were screened for age, for intention to undertake long-distance travel and for a number of other health issues relating to their risk and previous history of DVT.

▶ 'Volunteers were recruited by placing advertisements in local newspapers...'

▶ 'Passengers were included if they were over 50 years of age and intended to travel economy class with two sectors of at least 8 h duration within 6 weeks.'

▶ 'Volunteers were excluded from the study if they had...' (various exclusions)

Size of study groups

A total of 231 subjects were recruited (116 received stockings; 116 no stockings). This seems small, as a 10% DVT rate would give only 12 events, well short of our 50. So it is only adequate if the effect is extremely large.

See 'Volunteers and methods: Participants ' (DVT trial p 1485).

Allocation — Were the study groups comparable?

It is vital that the groups are matched as closely as possible in every way except for the intervention (or exposure or other indicator) being studied. If the groups are not comparable to begin with, then a difference in outcomes may be due to one of the non-matched characteristics (or confounding factors) rather than due to the intervention (or exposure or other indicator) under consideration. For example, ways in which groups could differ include:

▸ age

▸ sex

▸ smoker/non-smoker

▸ disease severity or stage

▸ other risk factors

▸ .... (there are many more).

The *most* important matching factors are those that predict the outcome of the condition, which is often most related to the severity of the illness.

Comparability of groups

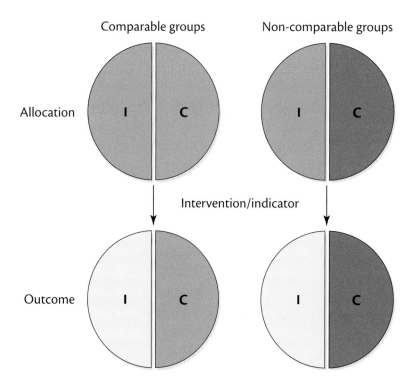

Methods to ensure that study groups are comparable vary according to the type of study. The ideal method is experimental (such as RCTs), where the researcher randomly allocates the subjects to groups — a process that must be very carefully managed to avoid bias that would lead to the groups not being comparable.

Steps in critical appraisal of primary research

Recruitment

Were the subjects representative of the target population?

Allocation or adjustment

Was the treatment allocation concealed before randomisation and were the groups comparable at the start of the trial?

Maintenance

Was the comparable status of the study groups maintained through equal management and adequate follow-up?

Measurement

Were the outcomes measured with:

blinded subjects and assessors, and/or

objective outcomes?

For observational studies, cohorts of subjects, or groups of cases, need to be matched with comparison cohorts or groups. Once again, this is a process that needs to be very carefully managed and often requires careful statistical adjustments to be made to ensure that the groups are comparable (but this is never completely possible, so randomization is preferred wherever feasible). These two approaches (allocation and adjustment) are briefly described below.

Allocation to groups

For experimental studies, once subjects have consented to take part in the trial, they are randomly allocated to either the control or intervention (or exposure/ indicator) group. However, randomisation can be done very well or rather badly. To be effective, the process used for randomisation must ensure that neither the trial subjects nor the investigators can influence the group each person ends up in ('allocation concealment'). This is because if either the practitioner or the subjects know which group each person is allocated to before they consent, selective allocation may occur and skew the groups. Similarly, if the subjects know which group they are in, this can also introduce bias in the reporting of outcomes (see discussion of 'Measurement' on pages 86–88).

Allocation concealment is best achieved by using a centralised computer allocation process. This method is usually used for large multicentre trials. For smaller trials, use of an independent person (such as the hospital pharmacist) and a sealed envelope system gives a satisfactory result.

Methods such as allocating alternate subjects to each group or handing out sealed envelopes are not as good because the allocation is not as well concealed.

Other allocation methods are sometimes used, including allocating subjects to groups on alternate days as they first come for treatment, or selecting subjects from databases, but these methods do not conceal allocation and are not truly randomised.

Whatever method is used for selection of subjects and group allocation, something unexpected can happen so it is important to check that the groups formed are really closely matched for as many characteristics as possible.

In order to fully conceal allocation, it may be necessary to give the subjects in the control group a placebo, or sham, treatment that is indistinguishable from the real thing. This also overcomes the problem of the placebo effect (see 'Measurement' on pages 86–88).

Adjustment for confounding

For observational studies, such as cohort studies and case-control studies, the subjects are not allocated to groups randomly and, in these cases, the way in which study groups are formed and matched become the critical quality issues. As perfect matching is almost never possible in non-randomised studies, statistical adjustments are needed to approximate comparability of the study groups. This issue is discussed further in Part 3 of this workbook, which includes an example of a critical appraisal of a cohort study to answer a prognosis question.

Allocation — Were the DVT trial study groups comparable?

Randomisation and concealment

The DVT trial is an experimental study in which the selected volunteers were allocated to either the stocking or no stocking (control) group. To assess whether the groups created were likely to be comparable (ie not biased), we need to ask whether the allocation was random and whether it was concealed from anyone who could influence the outcome.

The paper states:

▶ 'Volunteers were randomised *by sealed envelope* to one of two groups'

See 'Volunteers and methods: Randomisation' (DVT trial p 1486).

We know that envelopes are not always well concealed from clinicians or patients, so when study groups are allocated this way they can become skewed.

Characteristics of the study groups

Because the allocation was not fully concealed, we need to check that a good balance was achieved between the two groups. RCT papers usually include a table showing relevant characteristics of the study groups. The group characteristics table from the DVT trial is shown below. It indicates that females were more likely to be 'randomised' to the stocking group (and that this difference was statistically significant).

See 'Table 1' (DVT trial p1486).

	No stockings	Stockings
Number	**116**	**115**
Pre-study:		
Age	62 (56–68)	61 (56–66)
Females	61 (53%)	81 (70%)*
Varicose veins	41	45
Haemoglobin	142	140
During study:		
Hours flying	22	24
Days of stay	17	16

* $P < 0.01$

The importance of any differences between the study groups depends on the relationship of the differences to the outcome being studied, which should be discussed by the authors of the paper. In the case of the DVT trial the authors claimed that there is little evidence that women over 50 are more or less susceptible to venous thrombosis than men of the same age.

See 'Discussion' (DVT trial p 1488).

Maintenance — Was the comparable status of the study groups maintained through equal management and adequate follow-up?

Once comparable groups have been set up, it is important that they stay that way! That is, the management and follow-up of the groups should maintain the comparable status of the groups.

Equal management

The study groups should be managed so that the only difference between the groups is the factor being tested (for example, treatment with a specific drug or exposure to a specific risk factor, such as cigarette smoking). In comparative studies, this means that the control group should be treated exactly the same as the experimental group in every respect except for the factor being tested.

> ### Unequal treatment invalidates results
>
> In a trial of vitamin E in pre-term infants (1948), the vitamin treatment appeared to 'prevent' retrolental fibroplasia. However, this was not due to the vitamin itself but because the babies were on 100% oxygen and the treatment group babies were removed from the oxygen for frequent doses of vitamin, whereas the control babies remained in the oxygen.

Particular care also needs to be taken to use an identical measurement strategy for everyone (both the study and control groups) to avoid measurement error. This can occur, for example, if different equipment, different methods or different assessors are used to measure the outcomes for subjects in each study group.

Measurement error

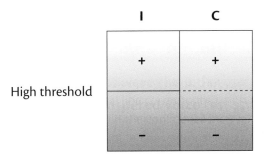

High threshold

Low threshold

Steps in critical appraisal of primary research

Recruitment

Were the subjects representative of the target population?

Allocation or adjustment

Was the treatment allocation concealed before randomisation and were the groups comparable at the start of the trial?

Maintenance

Was the comparable status of the study groups maintained through equal management and adequate follow-up?

Measurement

Were the outcomes measured with:

> **b**linded subjects and assessors, and/or
>
> **o**bjective outcomes?

Adequate follow-up

Inevitably, some subjects drop out, change groups or are variously lost to follow-up during a study. This is a serious problem because the remaining groups may no longer be comparable.

Therefore, this question is about checking that none of these things have happened. It involves checking that:

▶ subjects at the start = subjects at the end (that is, the majority of the subjects have been accounted for)

▶ subjects are analysed in the groups that they started out in (this is known as the 'intention-to-treat principle').

'Intention-to-treat principle'

Once a subject is randomised, he or she should be analysed in the group they are randomised to, even if they never receive treatment, discontinue the trial, or cross over to the other group.

The results can also be biased if the subjects are not followed up for long enough for relevant outcomes to be revealed in both groups. It is therefore important that the subjects are followed up until the relevant outcome occurs, or until death (for cohort studies).

Maintenance — Was the comparable status of the DVT trial groups maintained?

Management and measurement

Once the subjects had been allocated to the groups in the DVT trial, the subsequent pre-travel management, travel arrangements and measurement strategy were the same for both groups.

See 'Volunteers and methods: Investigators' (DVT trial pp1485–1486) and 'Evaluation' (p1486).

Follow-up of subjects

'Passengers reattended the Stamford Hospital within 48 h of their return flight.'

At this time, the passengers had an ultrasound examination for symptomless DVT and a blood test.

See 'Volunteers and methods: Evaluation' (DVT trial p 1486).

Losses to follow-up

Research papers reporting RCTs should include a flowchart showing the numbers of subjects and their progress through the trial. The DVT trial flowchart shows:

231 subjects were randomised (115 to stockings; 116 none)

200 were analysed; that is, 31 were lost to follow-up as follows:

▶ 27 unable to attend for subsequent ultrasound

▶ 2 were excluded from analysis because they were upgraded to business class

▶ 2 were excluded from analysis because they were taking anticoagulants.

How important were the losses?

Were they equally distributed?

▶ stockings: 15 lost (6 men; 9 women)

▶ no stockings: 16 lost (7 men, 9 women)

Did they have similar characteristics?

▶ No other information is provided about the characteristics of the lost subjects.

Analysis of results

'Haematological data were included in the analysis only when volunteers were examined before and after travel. All other analyses were done on an intention-to-treat basis, which included all randomised participants.'

See 'Trial profile' and 'Results' (DVT trial pp 1486 and 1487).

Measurement — Were the outcomes measured with blinded subjects and assessors and/or objective measures?

Even if the study groups have been randomly allocated or adjusted to ensure comparability at the start of the study, most subjects accounted for, relevant outcomes obtained and analysed in the starting groups, everything can still go pear shaped if the outcomes are not measured fairly!

Measurement error due to non-standardised measurements for the different groups in the study has already been discussed on page 83. However, the most common cause of serious problems with outcome measurements is 'measurement bias'. This bias reflects the human tendency to unfairly 'nudge' results in the direction that they predict the results should go.

If the subjects know which group they are in this may affect the way they behave in the trial, comply with the treatment regimen, report their symptoms and so on.

If the person who is making the measurement (outcome assessor) knows which group the subject is in, this can influence the way in which they record the results.

These biases can be overcome by using subjects and outcome assessors that are both 'blinded' to which groups the subjects are allocated to. A trial that is set up this way is called a 'double-blind' trial and the results of such a study are least likely to be biased.

A trial in which either the subjects or the outcome assessors are blinded to the group allocation, but not both, is called a single-blind study and the results are less reliable than for a double-blind study because of the increased potential for bias. A study in which neither the subjects nor the outcome assessors are blinded is the least reliable type of study of all because of the high potential for bias.

Of course, measurement bias will be significantly reduced if the outcomes measured are **objective** (such as weight) rather than subjective (such as feeling better). For highly objective measures, such as death or standardised machine-read laboratory measurements, assessors may not need to be blinded. But for subjective measurements, blinding is crucial. So even if the subjects and treating doctors or researchers cannot be blinded, the study should attempt to have the outcome assessors blind to which groups the subjects are in.

Steps in critical appraisal of primary research

Recruitment

Were the subjects representative of the target population?

Allocation or adjustment

Was the treatment allocation concealed before randomisation and were the groups comparable at the start of the trial?

Maintenance

Was the comparable status of the study groups maintained through equal management and adequate follow-up?

Measurement

Were the outcomes measured with:

> **b**linded subjects and assessors, and/or

> **o**bjective outcomes?

> **'Blinding'**
>
> **BEST** — *Double-blind trial*: subjects and investigators (outcome assessors) both unaware of group allocation
>
> **MODERATE** — *Single-blind trial*: either the subject or the investigators are unaware of group allocation
>
> **WORST** — *Not blinded*: subjects and investigators both aware of group allocation

Placebo effect

An common source of measurement bias for experimental studies is the so-called 'placebo effect'. This is the effect that is attributable to the expectation that a treatment will have an effect.

Placebo effect — Trial in patients with chronic severe itching

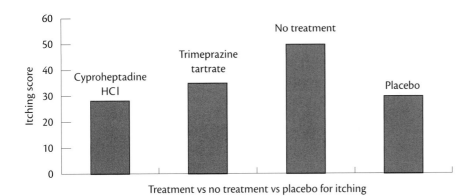

Thus, in a trial where a treatment is compared with no treatment, an effect (even quite a large one) may be due to the 'placebo effect', rather than to the effect of the treatment itself. This means that whenever it is practical to do so, the control group in an RCT should receive a placebo treatment that is indistinguishable from the real thing (eg a sugar pill, or sham procedure).

Measurement — Were the DVT trial outcomes measured with blinded subjects and assessors and/or objective measures?

Subjects

'Although the stockings were allocated randomly, the passengers were aware of the treatment' (ie were not blinded).

Using a 'placebo' stocking (a low-pressure stocking) would have been better as it would have blinded the subjects to which group they were in, thus reducing any tendency for the subjects in the two groups to behave differently during their flights.

See 'Volunteers and methods: Randomisation' (DVT trial p 1486).

Outcome assessors

'Most passengers removed their stockings on completion of their journey. The nurse removed the stockings from those passengers who had continued to wear them. A further duplex examination was then undertaken with the technician unaware of the group to which the volunteer had been randomised' (ie blinded)

The outcome measured in the DVT trial (symptomless DVT in the calf) was subject to some interpretation by the ultrasound technician, making blinding of the technicians an important quality issue for this trial.

See 'Volunteers and methods: Evaluation (DVT trial p 1486).

Question 3: What do the results mean?

When you have assessed the study using the above criteria, you may decide that it is not worth using it to inform your decision making any further. If you do decide that the study is suitable for further consideration (or, perhaps, if it is the only study available), the next stage is to turn to the results section and ask 'What do the results show and could they have been due to chance?'

Outcome measures

Results can be presented either as binary outcomes (which are also called dichotomous outcomes), that is, 'yes' or 'no' outcomes that either happen or don't happen, such as cancer, heart attack or death; or continuous outcomes, such as weight, height or the amount of cholesterol in blood.

Binary outcomes

Consider a study in which 15 out of 100 subjects (15% or 0.15) in the control group and 10 out of 100 subjects (10% or 0.10) in the treatment group died after 2 years of treatment. The results can be expressed in many ways as shown in the table on page 90.

Continuous outcomes

Continuous outcomes are measures that vary along a continuum (such as height, weight). The important measures are the group means. The difference between the treatment and control group means tells us how large or small the effect is.

Are the results real and relevant?

If the results of a study appear to show an effect, you will also need to work out if this is a real effect or one that is due to chance.

We can never determine the exact risk of a binary outcome in a population or the exact level of a continuous outcome. The best we can do is to estimate the true risk or level based on the sample of subjects in a trial. How do we know that the estimate from the study reflects the true population situation?

This is where statistics comes in and we will not go into the statistical methods used in detail here. Suffice to say that statistics provides two methods of assessing chance:

▶ *P*-values (hypothesis testing)

▶ confidence intervals (estimation).

Outcome measures for binary outcomes

Measure	Meaning	Example
Relative risk (RR) = risk of outcome in the treatment group/ risk of event in the control group	RR tells us how many times more likely it is that an event will occur in the treatment group relative to the control group RR = 1 means that there is no difference between the 2 groups RR < 1 means that the treatment reduces the risk of the event RR > 1 means that the treatment increases the risk of the event	RR = 0.1/0.15 = 0.67 Since this RR< 1, the treatment decreases the risk of death
Absolute risk reduction (ARR) = risk of event in the control group – risk of event in the treatment group (also known as the absolute risk difference)	ARR tells us the absolute difference in the rates of events between the two groups and gives an indication of the baseline risk and treatment effect ARR = 0 means that there is no difference between the 2 groups (thus, the treatment had no effect) ARR positive means that the treatment is beneficial ARR negative means that the treatment is harmful	ARR = 0.15 – 0.10 = 0.05 (5%) The absolute benefit of treatment is a 5% reduction in the death rate (ie there were 5 fewer deaths in the treatment group compared to the control group)
Relative risk reduction (RRR) = ARR/risk of event in control group (or 1 – RR)	RRR tells us the reduction in rate of the event in the treatment group relative to the rate in the control group **RRR is probably the most commonly reported measure of treatment effects**	RRR = 0.05/0.15 = 0.33 (33%) OR 1–0.67 = 0.33 (33%)
Number needed to treat (NNT) = 1/ARR	NNT tells us the number of patients we need to treat in order to prevent 1 bad event	NNT = 1/0.05 = 20 We would need to treat 20 people for 2 years in order to prevent 1 death

Note: Results are also often expressed as an 'odds ratio' (OR), where odds are a measure of probability rather than risk. However, the OR is approximately equal to RR. (See the 'Glossary' in Part 4 of this workbook for further information.)

P-values are a measure of the probability that a result is purely due to chance – so we want a low P-value suggesting that chance is an unlikely cause of the difference between groups. Scientific research is about testing a 'null hypothesis' (which means a hypothesis that there will not be an effect). If the result of the study (the point estimate) shows an effect (ie the null hypothesis appears unlikely), the P-value tells us the probability that this effect could be due simply to chance. If the P-value is low (usually less than 0.05), it means that the probability that the result was due to chance is also low (less than 5%); that is, it is a real effect (or a bias, which is why we need to critically appraise before looking at the P-value). An effect with a low P-value is called a 'statistically significant' result, which we shouldn't confuse with a clinically important result (which is explained below).

Confidence intervals (CIs) are generally more informative than P-values. They are an estimate of the range of values that are likely to include the real value. Usually CIs are quoted as 95% CIs, which means the range of values that have a 95% chance of including the real value. If the 95% CI for the difference between treatment and control groups is small and does not overlap the 'no effect' point (0 for a difference or 1 for a ratio), we can be pretty sure that the result is real (that is, with a P-value less than 0.05).

The more subjects that there are in the study, the narrower the CIs are likely to be and therefore larger studies give more reliable results than smaller studies. However, just how large the study needs to be to give a meaningful result depends on how rare the event being measured is. This basic rule of thumb is described in the paper by Glasziou and Doll ('Was the study big enough? Two café rules'), which is included in the 'Further reading' section of this workbook.

Statistical significance

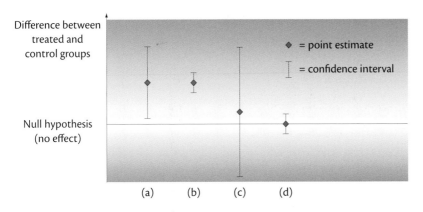

(a) Statistically significant result (P < 0.05) but low precision
(b) Statistically significant result (P < 0.05) with high precision
(c) Not statistically significant result (P > 0.05) with low precision
(d) Not statistically significant result (no effect) with high precision

However, an intervention can only be considered useful if the 95% CI includes clinically important treatment effects. An important distinction therefore needs to be made between statistical significance and clinical importance:

▶ statistical significance relates to the size of the effect and the 95% CI in relation to the null hypothesis

▶ clinical importance relates to the size of the effect and the 95% CI in relation to a minimum effect that would be considered to be clinically important.

For example, a reduction in a symptom may be measurable and statistically significant, but unless it is sufficient to avoid the need for medication or improve the quality of life of the patient, then it may not be considered clinically important.

Clinical importance

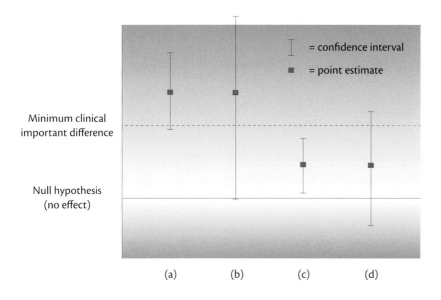

(a) Difference is statistically significant and clinically important
(b) Difference is not statistically significant but is clinically important
(c) Difference is statistically significant but not clinically important
(d) Difference is not statistically significant and not clinically important

What do the results of the DVT trial mean?

DVT in stocking group	= 0 [absolute risk (AR) = 0%]
DVT in control group	= 12 [AR = 12%]
Absolute risk reduction (ARR)	= 12% − 0%
	= 12%

The 95% CI for the ARR is not quoted in the paper, but we have calculated this to be 7–18%. Although the P-value is not quoted in the paper, this result is statistically significant because the CI does not overlap with 0 (which is the value of the ARR if there were no effect).

This means that this study shows that absolute benefit of wearing stockings is a 12% reduction in symptomless DVTs.

Number needed to treat (NNT) to avoid one case of DVT = 1/0.12 = 8

See 'Results', (DVT trial p1487).

Summary of critical appraisal of the DVT trial

PICO

The PICO of the DVT trial closely matches our clinical question about whether wearing elastic stockings on long-haul flights reduces the risk of DVT.

Internal validity

Recruitment

In the DVT trial, subjects were initially recruited on a volunteer basis. Inclusion/exclusion criteria ensured that the recruited subjects were representative of the population of interest (over 50 years of age, travelling long distance by economy class, no previous history of DVT, etc). Although not a very large study, the numbers of subjects (approximately 100 subjects per group) was sufficient to provide a representative sample (and hence statistically meaningful results).

R

Allocation

Group allocation was random but the method used (sealed envelope) was not a very effective method for eliminating allocation bias. The subjects knew which group they were in.

A

Due either to allocation bias (were women more prepared to wear elastic stockings?) or to other factors, there was a statistically significant difference in sex ratio between the groups. The groups were well matched for other factors.

Maintenance

Once allocated to groups, all subjects were managed equally, relevant outcomes were measured using the same methodology for both groups and there were only a few losses to follow-up.

M

Measurement

M

▶ **B**linding — the outcome assessors (ultrasonographers) were generally not aware of which study groups the subjects were in (ie were blinded). However, the subjects knew which groups they were in and there was no placebo treatment so that a difference in behaviour during the flights between the two groups could not be ruled out.

b

▶ **O**bjectivity — the outcome measure was subject to some interpretation by the ultrasound technician (ie not objective).

o

Overall (internal validity): The trial was moderately well conducted but had some methodological flaws that could have affected the outcomes.

Results

The results showed a large difference between the treated and control groups, which was statistically significant (because the CIs did not overlap with zero).

Absolute risk reduction (ARR)　　= 0.12 (12%; 95%CI, 7% to 18%)
NNT　　= 1/0.12 = 8

Conclusion

While the results show a reduction in symptomless DVT in passengers on long-haul flights, the study had some design flaws that would warrant further investigation of this issue.

While an NNT of 8 is impressive, the importance of this remains a matter of clinical judgment about the consequences, such as the small number that may become symptomatic, the even smaller number of DVTs that may cause pulmonary embolism, and the uncertain number of people who will go on to develop postphlebitic syndrome some years in the future. That is a difficult judgment. However, you may be interested to know that the authors of this workbook all wear elastic stockings on long flights (although this is partly for increased comfort and to reduce ankle swelling).

Frequency and prevention of symptomless deep-vein thrombosis in long-haul flights: a randomised trial

John H Scurr, Samuel J Machin, Sarah Bailey-King, Ian J Mackie, Sally McDonald, Philip D Coleridge Smith

Summary

Background The true frequency of deep-vein thrombosis (DVT) during long-haul air travel is unknown. We sought to determine the frequency of DVT in the lower limb during long-haul economy-class air travel and the efficacy of graduated elastic compression stockings in its prevention.

Methods We recruited 89 male and 142 female passengers over 50 years of age with no history of thromboembolic problems. Passengers were randomly allocated to one of two groups: one group wore class-I below-knee graduated elastic compression stockings, the other group did not. All the passengers made journeys lasting more than 8 h per flight (median total duration 24 h), returning to the UK within 6 weeks. Duplex ultrasonography was used to assess the deep veins before and after travel. Blood samples were analysed for two specific common gene mutations, factor V Leiden (FVL) and prothrombin G20210A (PGM), which predispose to venous thromboembolism. A sensitive D-dimer assay was used to screen for the development of recent thrombosis.

Findings 12/116 passengers (10%; 95% CI 4·8–16·0%) developed symptomless DVT in the calf (five men, seven women). None of these passengers wore elastic compression stockings, and two were heterozygous for FVL. Four further patients who wore elastic compression stockings, had varicose veins and developed superficial thrombophlebitis. One of these passengers was heterozygous for both FVL and PGM. None of the passengers who wore class-I compression stockings developed DVT (95% CI 0–3·2%).

Interpretation We conclude that symptomless DVT might occur in up to 10% of long-haul airline travellers. Wearing of elastic compression stockings during long-haul air travel is associated with a reduction in symptomless DVT.

Lancet 2001; **357**: 1485–89
See Commentary page 1461

Introduction

Every year the number of passengers travelling over long distances by air increases. Physicians working close to major airports have seen individual cases presenting with thromboembolic problems after air travel.[1-3] Results of retrospective clinical series[4-6] suggest that up to 20% of patients presenting with thromboembolism have undertaken recent air travel. Ferrari et al[7] reported a strong association between deep-vein thrombosis (DVT) and long travel (>4 h) in a case-control study, although only a quarter of his patients with DVT travelled by air. Kraaijenhagen and colleagues[8] looked at travel in the previous 4 weeks in patients presenting with DVT. They concluded that travelling times of more than 5 h were not associated with increased risk of DVT. The true frequency of this problem remains unknown and controversial. Episodes of DVT can arise without any symptom. Less than half the patients with symptomless DVT will develop symptoms, and only a few of those go on to have a clinically detectable pulmonary embolism.[9,10] In surgical series, a link between symptomless DVT, symptomatic DVT, and pulmonary embolism has been established.[11,12] Patients undergoing surgical procedures are assessed for risk, and appropriate prophylaxis is implemented.[13] We undertook a randomised controlled trial to assess the overall frequency of DVT in long-haul airline passengers and the efficacy of a class-I elastic compression stocking for the duration of the flight.

Volunteers and methods

Participants

Volunteers were recruited by placing advertisements in local newspapers and travel shops, and by press releases. The Aviation Health Institute referred many of the volunteers initially screened for this study, which took place in the Vascular Institute at the Stamford Hospital, London, UK. Passengers were included if they were over 50 years of age and intended to travel economy class with two sectors of at least 8 h duration within 6 weeks. Passengers were invited to undergo preliminary screening, which included an examination and completion of a medical questionnaire about previous illnesses and medication. Volunteers were excluded from the study if they had had episodes of venous thrombosis, were taking anticoagulants, regularly wore compression stockings, had cardiorespiratory problems, or had any other serious illness, including malignant disease. The study was approved by Stamford Hospital ethics committee. Volunteers who gave informal written consent were included in the study.

Investigators

Volunteers who were eligible for inclusion were investigated by duplex ultrasonography (General Electric LOGIQ 700, GE Medical Systems, Waukesha, USA) to detect evidence of previous venous thrombosis. The lower limbs were assessed by two technicians skilled in assessment of venous problems. Examinations were done with volunteers standing. To assess the competence of deep and superficial veins the technicians manually

Department of Surgery (J H Scurr FRCS, P D Coleridge Smith FRCS) **and Department of Haematology** (Prof S J Machin FRCP, I J Mackie PhD, S McDonald BSc), **Royal Free and University College Medical School, London, UK; and Stamford Hospital, London, UK** (S Bailey-King RCN)

Correspondence to: Mr J H Scurr, Lister Hospital, Chelsea Bridge Road, London SW1W 8RH, UK
(e-mail: medleg@mailbox.co.uk)

Reproduced from *The Lancet* with permission from Elsevier.

compressed the calf and measured the duration of reverse flow by colour or pulsed doppler sonography. Venous reflux was defined as duration of reverse flow exceeding 0·5 s. The presence of current or previous venous thrombosis was assessed from the B-mode image, colour flow mapping, and compression assessment of veins during B-mode imaging. Passengers who had evidence of previous thrombosis were excluded.

In the first 30 volunteers, ultrasound examination was undertaken 2 weeks before air travel and again within 2 days of the start of the first flight to provide a control interval in which occurrence of spontaneous DVT could be assessed in this population. No acute DVT was detected during this period. The logistics of the study made it difficult for passengers to attend Stamford Hospital on two occasions before travel and this part of the investigation was abandoned in the remaining volunteers. All subsequent volunteers were screened once before they travelled.

Blood was taken from all participants before travel for a series of haemostatic tests. Full blood and platelet counts were done on a routine cell counter. We used the Dimertest Gold EIA assay (Agen Biomedical Ltd, Acacia Ridge, Australia) to measure D-dimer. We took the upper 95% confidence limit of normal value as 120 pg/L. We used routine PCR techniques for identification of the factor V Leiden and prothrombin G20210A gene mutations.

Randomisation

Volunteers were randomised by sealed envelope to one of two groups. The control group received no specific additional treatment; the other group was given class-I (German Hohenstein compression standard; 20–30 mm Hg) below-knee elastic compression stockings (Mediven Travel; Medi UK Ltd, Hereford, UK). Participants were advised to put on the stockings before the start of travel and to remove the stockings after arrival for every flight by which they travelled. Although the stockings were allocated randomly, the passengers were aware of the treatment. Passengers arranged their own air travel. There was no collaboration with the airlines, although two passengers were upgraded from economy to business class.

Evaluation

Passengers reattended the Stamford Hospital within 48 h of their return flight. They were interviewed by a research nurse and completed a questionnaire inquiring about: duration of air travel, wearing of stockings, symptoms in the lower limbs, and illnesses and medication taken during their trip. Most passengers removed their stockings on completion of their journey. The nurse removed the stockings from those passengers who had continued to wear them. A further duplex examination was then undertaken with the technician unaware of the group to which the volunteer had been randomised. Another blood sample was taken for repeat D-dimer assay. In passengers for whom clinically significant abnormalities of the lower limb veins were detected on duplex ultrasonography, including calf vein thrombosis, the volunteers' general practitioners were notified in writing so that treatment could be arranged.

Statistics

Because of insufficient published data we could not pre-calculate sample size. Since the investigation was intended as a pilot study, we chose a total of 200 passengers. Recruitment was continued until 100 volunteers had been investigated in each group. A finding

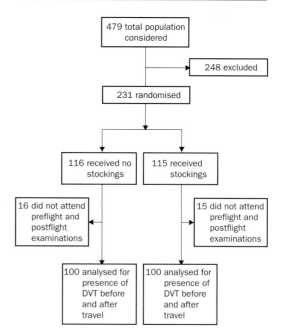

Trial profile

of no case of venous thrombosis in this number of passengers would have resulted in a 95% CI for the rate of DVT of 0–2%. To measure a thrombotic event occurring in 2% or fewer passengers would require a very large study, and the low frequency would have limited implications for air travellers. Data were analysed by contingency tables and calculation of the differences in proportions, and 95% CIs by a computer program (CIA version 1.1, 1989, BMA Publishers, London, UK). We used median and interquartile range for haematological data since data were not normally distributed. Haematological data were included in the analysis only when volunteers were examined before and after travel. All other analyses were done on an intention-to-treat basis, which included all randomised participants.

Results

Volunteers were excluded before randomisation if they did not fulfil the entry requirements or could not attend hospital for investigation both before and after travel (figure). Thus, 231 of 479 volunteers were randomised. 27 passengers were unable to attend for subsequent ultrasound investigation because of ill-health (three), change of travel plans, or inability to keep appointments (24). Two who

	No stockings	Stockings
Number	116	115
Age (years)	62 (56–68)	61 (56–66)
Number of women (%)	61 (53%)	81 (70%)
Number with varicose veins	41	45
Days of stay	17 (13–32)	16 (13–27)
Hours flying time	22 (18–36)	24 (19–35)
Haemoglobin (g/L)	142 (133–149)	140 (133–147)
WBC (×10⁹/L)	5·9 (5·0–7·3)	6·0 (5·0–6·9)
Packed cell volume	0·44 (0·42–0·47)	0·44 (0·41–0·46)
Platelets (×10⁹/L)	240 (206–272)	242 (219–290)
Number FVL positive	7	4
Number PGM positive	1	3

Median (interquartile range) shown, unless otherwise indicated. WBC=white blood cells. FVL=factor V Leiden. PGM=prothrombin gene mutation.

Table 1: **Characteristics of study groups**

Reproduced with permission.

	DVT	No DVT	SVT	No SVT
Number	12	188	4	196
Number of women	7	117	4	120
Age (years)	67 (58–68)	62 (55–68)	67 (64–70)	62 (55–68)
Days of stay	18 (8–21)	16 (13–27)	18 (16–21)	16 (13–26)
Hours flying time	21 (17–25)	24 (18–27)	28 (25–33)	24 (18–35)
Haemoglobin (g/L)	142 (132–146)	140 (133–148)	130 (125–133)	140 (133–148)
WBC ($\times10^9$/L)	6·1 (5·7–7·0)	6·0 (5·0–7·1)	6·3 (5·6–6·8)	6·0 (5·0–7·2)
Packed cell volume	0·44 (0·42–0·47)	0·44 (0·42–0·47)	0·40 (0·39–0·40)	0·44 (0·42–0·47)
Platelets ($\times10^9$/L)	240 (206–272)	244 (216–285)	264 (237–236)	241 (214–286)
Number FVL positive	2	9	1	10
Number PGM positive	0	4	1	3
Preflight D-dimer (pg/L)*	44,45,54,66	ND	33,58	ND
Postflight D-dimer (pg/L)	33,41,54,59,63,91	ND	36,93	ND
Stockings	0	100	4	96

Volunteers grouped according to presence of symptomless deep vein thrombosis (DVT) and superficial thrombophlebitis (SVT). Median (interquartile range) shown, unless otherwise indicated. WBC=white blood cells. FVL=factor V Leiden. PGM=prothrombin gene mutation. ND=not detectable (below the limit of sensitivity of the assay, 32 pg/L). *D-dimer values are those individual values greater than 32 pg/L, all other passengers had concentrations less than 32 pg/L.

Table 2: **Age and haematological data in 200 passengers examined before and after air travel**

were upgraded to business class and two taking anticoagulants were also excluded. A similar number of men and women were excluded in the two groups: six and nine in the stocking group and seven and nine in the no stocking group, respectively. The remaining 200 passengers were invesigated before and after long-haul economy air travel. None of the 31 volunteers who were excluded after randomsiation underwent follow-up duplex ultrasound examination.

The characteristics of the two groups were closely matched, but by chance a greater proportion of women were included in the stocking group (table 1). Table 2 shows results of haematological investigations. After air travel, 12 (10%; 95% CI 4·8–16·0%) passengers not wearing elastic stockings had developed symptomless DVT in the calf that were detected on duplex ultrasound examination. None of the 115 passengers (CI 0–3·2%) wearing compression stockings had DVT. A further four people all of whom were wearing compression stockings, developed superficial thrombophlebitis in varicose veins (3%; 1·0–8·7%). None of the no-stockings-group developed superficial thrombophelbitis (0–3·1%). Four of the patients with symptomless DVT were given low-molecular-weight heparin subcutaneosuly for 5 days and were referred to their general practitioner for further treatment. The remaining eight were asked to take aspirin, referred to their general practitioner, and advised to undergo a further scan and receive treatment if appropriate. General practitioners were kept informed of these developments. The four passengers with superficial thrombophlebitis received treatment, one with aspirin and three with a non-steroidal anti-inflammatory drug (diclofenac).

14 (7%) of the 200 participants examined both before and after travel, were heterozygous for either factor V Leiden (11) or prothrombin gene mutation (four). One person had both gene mutations and had an episode of thrombophlebitis. Two passengers with symptomless DVT were factor V Leiden positive. The full blood count, platelet count, and D-dimer assays provided no prognostic information.

The before and after travel questionnaires were examined to identify concomitant medication, including that begun during air travel (table 3). Only two passengers took drugs in addition to their usual medication. Most drugs were evenly distributed in the two groups, although there was a trend towards more patients taking hormone replacement therapy in the stocking than in the non-stocking group (percentage difference 8%,CI −1 to 17%). Several volunteers took aspirin as part of their regular medication.

Discussion

About one in ten passengers not wearing elastic compression stockings developed symptomless DVT after airline travel, which is a surprisingly large proportion of the study group. The passengers were all aged more than 50 years and undertook long journeys by air (median 24 h), both of which are factors that could increase the risk of thrombosis. As far as we are aware no other workers have undertaken such a prospective study.

Other investigators[14] have shown postoperative symptomless DVT (detected by radio-fibrinogen scanning) in about 30% of general surgical patients in whom no prophylactic measure was applied. We accept that symptomless calf vein thrombosis is probably not a major risk to health, but the approach might be useful in future interventional studies. Published clinical series have recorded DVTs detected after investigation of calf symptoms. They showed that 10–20% of isolated calf vein thromboses extend to more proximal veins.[15,16] Pulmonary embolism can arise in about 10% of patients presenting with isolated calf vein thrombosis.[15,17] However, patients presenting with symptomatic calf vein thrombosis often have recognised predisposing factors such as malignant disease or thrombophilia.[15,16] We excluded patients with a history of serious illness or previous thrombotic episodes and all those with post-thrombotic vein damage on duplex ultrasonography. We believe that the thrombi detected in our study were attributable to long-haul air travel. Environmental changes that take place during long-haul air travel may provoke calf vein thrombosis. Once the journey has been completed these factors no longer apply, allowing spontaneous resolution of calf vein thromboses without complication in most cases.

In our study no symptomless DVT was detected in the stocking group. In hospital practice there is evidence that graduated compression stockings are effective at reducing the risk of DVT after surgical treatment.[18] Our findings strongly suggest that stockings also protect against

	Number of participants	
	No stockings	Stockings
Aspirin	9	11
Hormone replacement therapy	8	16
Thyroxine	6	6
Antihypertensives, including diuretics	10	12
Antipeptic ulcer drugs	8	3

*Includes additions to usual drugs.

Table 3: **All drugs taken by volunteers who attended for examination before and after air travel***

Reproduced with permission

97

symptomless DVT after air travel. However, four passengers with varicose veins developed superficial thrombophlebitis while wearing stockings. In all four, thrombophlebitis occurred in varicose veins in the knee region which were compressed by the upper edge of the stocking.

The prothrombotic gene mutations that we investigated are together present in about 10% of European populations. The combined prevalence of these abnormalities was 7% in our volunteers, but 19% in those developing superficial or deep venous thrombosis. These data should be regarded with caution, in view of the small number of people we studied.

D-dimer, a specific degradation product of cross-linked fibrin, measured by a sensitive EIA procedure, is a useful diagnostic aid in detection of venous thromboembolism.[19] Failure to detect raised concentrations of D-dimer in passengers with positive ultrasound scans might be related to the short half-life of D-dimer (about 6 h), combined with the long (up to 48 h) time of blood sampling on return from travel. This interval between completion of the final leg of air travel and testing may have affected the usefulness of the test. Additionally, in all volunteers who developed symptomless DVT, the thrombus arose only in calf veins which would also result in a modest rise in plasma D-dimer.

Ferrari and co-workers[7] have also shown an association between travel and developments of DVT, but only a quarter of their patients with DVT had travelled by air. Although Kraaijenhagen and colleagues[8] recorded no association of DVT with travel, many of their airline passengers have flown for less than 5 h. These case-control studies also indicate that DVT related to air travel is not a major healthcare problem, perhaps because only a small proportion of the population undertakes long-haul journeys at any time. These investigators included people with several potential confounding factors such as previous venous thrombosis, malignant disease, and recent surgery, whereas we excluded such individuals. Bendz et al[20] simulated long-haul flights in a hypobaric chamber and noted substantially increased plasma markers of thrombosis in volunteers exposed to reduced ambient pressure. A major drawback was that they did not have a control group. However, their findings suggest a possible additional mechanism for thrombosis after air travel. We measured D-dimer values but, because of the study design, we could not show an association with the development of symptomless DVT.

We accept that our method of recruitment was not ideal, although we did exclude individuals at highest risk. We were concerned that because of their interest in the problem some of the volunteers may have taken steps to reduce the occurrence of venous thrombosis—ie, by being active during the flight and drinking more fluids. We could not assess the effect that participation in the study had on the behaviour of volunteers while aboard the aircraft. These factors would have applied equally to both our study groups. Whether leg exercises, walking, or drinking water prevent thrombotic events after airline travel remains to be established.

The randomisation procedure was not stratified or miminised for any factor, since we regarded this study as a pilot investigation, which resulted in even distribution between the study groups for most factors. Volunteers with the most important predisposition to DVT—a previous history of evidence of DVT—were excluded, ensuring that no bias resulted from this factor.[21] However, the stocking group contained more women than men (table 1). There is little evidence that women are more or less susceptible than men to venous thrombosis in the age group we investigated.[22] After airline travel, symptomless DVT was more-or-less evenly distributed between men and women (five of 55 men and seven of 61 women, table 3) in the non-stocking group.

We used duplex ultrasonography to detect symptomless DVT. Venography was judged unethical in symptomless volunteers. Others have shown[23,24] that duplex ultrasonography is a reliable method of detecting calf vein thrombosis, as well as proximal vein thrombosis, in symptom-free patients. In a series of studies the reliability of duplex ultrasonography in the diagnosis of calf vein thrombosis has been compared with venography.[25-29] The main failing of duplex ultrasonography is that it may underestimate the true frequency of calf vein thrombosis, but it has a specificity of 79–99%. Our data may have underestimated the true rate of calf vein thrombosis by as much as 30%. The fact that some individuals wore compression stockings until shortly before the post-travel examination is unlikely to have affected the sensitivity of the test. The most important factors determining the reliability of this examination are whether it is technically possible to image the deep veins and the presence of post-thrombotic vein damage.[28] All volunteers with post-thrombotic appearance on ultrasonography were excluded from this investigation and none of our participants had severe calf swelling, which would have prevented adequate images of the calf veins being obtained. We believe that the frequency of symptomless DVT that we recorded is reliable.

Contributors
John Scurr, Samuel Machin, Ian Mackie and Philip Coleridge Smith designed the study. John Scurr and Sarah Bailey-King recruited volunteers. Day to day conduct of study, record keeping and assessment of volunteers and clincial data analysis was the responsibility of Sarah Bailey-King. Ian Mackie and Sally McDonald did the haematological investigations. Overall analysis of data was by John Scurr and Philip Coleridge Smith, and statistical analysis by Philip Coleridge Smith. The writing committee consisted of John Scurr, Samuel Machin, and Philip Coleridge Smith.

Acknowledgments
We thank staff of Stamford Hospital for providing nursing and administrative support for this study, and for agreeing to undertake the duplex ultrasound examinations. Medi UK Ltd supplied the stockings worn by volunteers and provided a grant to cover the costs of the haematological examinations.
John Scurr is presently evaluating a device for increasing blood flow through the legs. He has spoken on behalf of the manufacturer to endorse this product. This research began after the current paper was submitted to *The Lancet*.

References
1   Patel A, Fuchs GJ. Air travel and thromboembolic complications after percutaneous nephrolithotomy for staghorn stone. *J Endourol* 1998; **12:** 51–53.
2   Milne R. Venous thromboembolism and travel: is there an association? *J R Coll Phys Lond* 1992; **26:** 47–49.
3   Sahiar F, Mohler SR. Economy class syndrome. *Aviat Space Environ Med* 1994; **65:** 957–60.
4   Nissen P. The so-called "economy class" syndrome or travel thrombosis. *Vasa* 1997; **26:** 239–46.
5   Ribier G, Zizka V, Cysique J, Donatien Y, Glaudon G, Ramialison C. Venous thromboembolic complications following air travel. Retrospective study of 40 cases recorded in Martinique. *Rev Med Intern* 1997; **18:** 601–04.
6   Eklof B, Kistner RL, Masuda EM, Sonntag BV, Wong HP. Venous thromboembolism in association with prolonged air travel. *Dermatol Surg* 1996; **22:** 637–41.
7   Ferrari E, Chevallier T, Chapelier A, Baudouy M. Travel is a risk factor for venous thromboembolic disease: a case-control study. *Chest* 1999; **115:** 440–44.

Reproduced with permission

8 Kraaijenhagen RA, Haverkamp D, Koopman MMW, Prandoni P, Piovella F, Büller H. Travel and the risk of venous thrombosis. *Lancet* 2000; **356:** 1492–93.

9 Kakkar VV, Howe CT, Flanc C, Clarke MB. Natural history of postoperative deep-vein thrombosis. *Lancet* 1969; **2:** 230–32.

10 Negus D, Pinto DJ. Natural history of postoperative deep-vein thrombosis. *Lancet* 1969; **2:** 645.

11 Dalen JE, Alpert JS. Natural history of pulmonary embolism. *Prog Cardiovasc Dis* 1975; **17:** 259–70.

12 Coon WW. Epidemiology of venous thromboembolism. *Ann Surg* 1977; **186:** 149–64.

13 THRIFT Consensus Group. Risk of and prophylaxis for venous thromboembolism in hospital patients. Thromboembolic Risk Factors. *BMJ* 1992; **305:** 567–74.

14 Collins R, Scrimgeour A, Yusuf S, Peto R. Reduction in fatal pulmonary embolism and venous thrombosis by perioperative administration of subcutaneous heparin. Overview of results of randomized trials in general, orthopaedic, and urologic surgery. *N Engl J Med* 1988; **318:** 1162–73.

15 Kazmers A, Groehn H, Meeker C. Acute calf vein thrombosis: outcomes and implications. *Am Surg* 1999; **65:** 1124–27.

16 O'Shaughnessy AM, Fitzgerald DE. The value of duplex ultrasound in the follow-up of acute calf vein thrombosis. *Int Angiol* 1997; **16:** 142–46.

17 Meissner MH, Caps MT, Bergelin RO, Manzo RA, Strandness DE Jr. Early outcome after isolated calf vein thrombosis. *J Vasc Surg* 1997; **26:** 749–56.

18 Colditz GA, Tuden RL, Oster G. Rates of venous thrombosis after general surgery: combined results of randomised clinical trials. *Lancet* 1986; **2:** 143–46.

19 Bounameaux H, de Moerloose P, Perrier A, Reber G. Plasma measurement of D-dimer as a diagnostic aid in suspected venous thromboembolism: an overview. *Thromb Haemost* 1994; **71:** 1–6.

20 Bendz B, Rostrup M, Sevre K, Andersen T, Sandset PM. Association between acute hypobaric hypoxia and activation of coagulation in human beings. *Lancet* 2000; **356:** 1657–58.

21 Nicolaides AN, Irving D. Clinical factors and the risk of deep vein thrombosis. In: Nicolaides AN, ed. Thromboembolism: aetiology, advances in prevention and management. Lancaster: MTP, 1975: 193–203.

22 Kniffin WD Jr, Baron JA, Barrett J, Birkmeyer JD, Anderson FA Jr. The epidemiology of diagnosed pulmonary embolism and deep venous thrombosis in the elderly. *Arch Intern Med* 1994; **154:** 861–66.

23 Robinson KS, Anderson DR, Gross M, et al. Accuracy of screening compression ultrasonography and clinical examination for the diagnosis of deep vein thrombosis after total hip or knee arthroplasty. *Can J Surg* 1998; **41:** 368–73.

24 Cornuz J, Pearson SD, Polak JF. Deep venous thrombosis: complete lower extremity venous US evaluation in patients without known risk factors—outcome study. *Radiology* 1999; **211:** 637–41.

25 Westrich GH, Allen ML, Tarantino SJ, et al. Ultrasound screening for deep venous thrombosis after total knee arthroplasty. 2-year reassessment. *Clin Orthop* 1998; **356:** 125–33.

26 Forbes K, Stevenson AJ. The use of power Doppler ultrasound in the diagnosis of isolated deep venous thrombosis of the calf. *Clin Radiol* 1998; **53:** 752–54.

27 Mantoni M, Strandberg C, Neergaard K, et al. Triplex US in the diagnosis of asymptomatic deep venous thrombosis. *Acta Radiol* 1997; **38:** 327–31.

28 Robertson PL, Goergen SK, Waugh JR, Fabiny RP. Colour-assisted compression ultrasound in the diagnosis of calf deep venous thrombosis. *Med J Aust* 1995; **163:** 515–18.

29 Krunes U, Teubner K, Knipp H, Holzapfel R. Thrombosis of the muscular calf veins-reference to a syndrome which receives little attention. *Vasa* 1998; **27:** 172–75.

Reproduced with permission

Rapid critical appraisal of your own primary study for an intervention question

Now you can critically appraise primary research studies for your intervention question that you found during your earlier search session. Remember that the best type of primary research for an intervention question is an RCT.

If you prefer, you can appraise the article on immunisation of infants that is included at the end of this section.[1]

For your chosen article, work through the critical appraisal sheet on the next few pages and then:

(a) decide whether the internal validity of the study is sufficient to allow firm conclusions (all studies have some flaws; but are these flaws bad enough to discard the study?)

(b) if the study is sufficiently valid, look at and interpret the results — what is the relevance or size of the effects of the intervention?

---

1   Since this study was published in 2000, a larger study of needle length has been published. However, we have retained the 2000 study for the purpose of this exercise.

Rapid critical appraisal of an RCT

Step 1: What question did the study ask?

Population/problem: ....

Intervention: ....

Comparison: ....

Outcome(s): ....

Step 2: How well was the study done? (internal validity)

<table>
<tr><td colspan="2">Recruitment — Were the subjects representative?</td></tr>
<tr><td>What is best?</td><td>Where do I find the information?</td></tr>
<tr><td>Do we know what group of patients this is (setting, inclusion/exclusion criteria)? Ideally, the subjects should be consecutive (or sometimes random), but the proportion of eligible patients who consent and are included should be known.</td><td>Early in the Methods should tell you how patients were selected for the study.</td></tr>
<tr><td colspan="2">This paper: Yes ☐   No ☐   Unclear ☐   Comment: ....</td></tr>
<tr><td colspan="2">Allocation — Was the allocation randomised and concealed....?</td></tr>
<tr><td>What is best?</td><td>Where do I find the information?</td></tr>
<tr><td>Centralised computer randomisation is ideal and often used in multicentre trials. Smaller trials may use an independent person (eg the hospital pharmacist) to 'police' the randomisation.</td><td>The Methods should tell you how patients were allocated to groups and whether or not randomisation was concealed. The authors should describe how the process was 'policed' or if there is some mention of masking (eg placebos with the same appearance or a sham therapy).</td></tr>
<tr><td colspan="2">This paper: Yes ☐   No ☐   Unclear ☐   Comment: ....</td></tr>
<tr><td colspan="2">.......... so that the groups were comparable at the start of the trial?</td></tr>
<tr><td>What is best?</td><td>Where do I find the information?</td></tr>
<tr><td>If the randomisation process worked (that is, achieved comparable groups) the groups should be similar. The more similar the groups, the better it is. There should be some indication of whether differences between groups are statistically significant (ie P-values).</td><td>The Results should have a table of 'Baseline characteristics' comparing the randomised groups on a number of variables that could affect the outcome (age, risk factors etc). If not, there may be a description of group similarity in the first paragraphs of the Results section.</td></tr>
<tr><td colspan="2">This paper: Yes ☐   No ☐   Unclear ☐   Comment: ....</td></tr>
</table>

Maintenance — Did the groups have equal co-interventions...?	
What is best?	**Where do I find the information?**
Apart from the intervention the patients in the different groups should be treated exactly the same (eg with respect to additional treatments or tests, measurements).	Look in the **Methods** for the precise protocol followed for each groups (such as follow-up schedule, permitted additional treatments) and in **Results** for any further information.
This paper: Yes ☐ No ☐ Unclear ☐ Comment:	

.... and was there adequate follow up?	
What is best?	**Where do I find the information?**
Losses to follow-up should be minimal – preferably less than 20%. Patients should also be analysed in the groups to which they were randomised – 'intention-to-treat analysis'.	The **Results** section should say how many patients were randomised and how many patients were actually included in the analysis. Sometimes a flowchart is given (but if not, try to draw one yourself).
This paper: Yes ☐ No ☐ Unclear ☐ Comment:	

Measurement — Were the subjects and assessors kept 'blind' to which treatment was being received and/or were the measures objective?	
What is best?	**Where do I find the information?**
For *objective* outcomes (eg death) blinding is less critical, but for *subjective* outcomes (eg symptoms or function) then blinding the outcome assessor is critical.	The **Methods** section should describe how the outcome was assessed and whether the assessor/s were aware of the patients' treatment.
This paper: Yes ☐ No ☐ Unclear ☐ Comment:	

Step 3: What do the results mean?

What measure was used and how large was the treatment effect?	
NNT (= 1/ARR)	
Could the effect have been due to chance?	
P-value	Confidence interval (CI)

Conclusion

Internal validity   ....

Results   ....

Effect of needle length on incidence of local reactions to routine immunisation in infants aged 4 months: randomised controlled trial

Linda Diggle, Jonathan Deeks

Abstract

Objective To compare rates of local reactions associated with two needle sizes used to administer routine immunisations to infants.

Design Randomised controlled trial.

Setting Routine immunisation clinics in eight general practices in Buckinghamshire.

Participants Healthy infants attending for third primary immunisation due at 16 weeks of age: 119 infants were recruited, and 110 diary cards were analysed.

Interventions Immunisation with 25 gauge, 16 mm, orange hub needle or 23 gauge, 25 mm, blue hub needle.

Main outcome measures Parental recordings of redness, swelling, and tenderness for three days after immunisation.

Results Rate of redness with the longer needle was initially two thirds the rate with the smaller needle (relative risk 0.66 (95% confidence interval 0.45 to 0.99), P = 0.04), and by the third day this had decreased to a seventh (relative risk 0.13 (0.03 to 0.56), P = 0.0006). Rate of swelling with the longer needle was initially about a third that with the smaller needle (relative risk 0.39 (0.23 to 0.67), P = 0.0002), and this difference remained for all three days. Rates of tenderness were also lower with the longer needle throughout follow up, but not significantly (relative risk 0.60 (0.29 to 1.25), P = 0.17).

Conclusions Use of 25 mm needles significantly reduced rates of local reaction to routine infant immunisation. On average, for every five infants vaccinated, use of the longer needle instead of the shorter needle would prevent one infant from experiencing any local reaction. Vaccine manufacturers should review their policy of supplying the shorter needle in vaccine packs.

Introduction

As part of the UK childhood immunisation schedule, infants routinely receive diphtheria, pertussis, and tetanus (DPT) vaccine and *Haemophilus influenzae* type b (Hib) vaccine at 2, 3, and 4 months.[1] Nationally available guidelines advise practitioners to administer primary vaccines to infants by deep subcutaneous or intramuscular injection using either a 25 or 23 gauge needle but give no recommendation regarding needle length.[1] The question of optimum needle length for infant immunisation has not previously been addressed in Britain, despite calls from nurses for evidence on which to base immunisation practice. We conducted a randomised controlled trial of the two needle sizes currently used by UK practitioners to determine whether needle size affects the incidence of redness, swelling, and tenderness.

Participants and methods

Participants

Eight of 11 general practices approached in Buckinghamshire agreed to participate in the study. Practice nurses recruited healthy infants attending routine immunisation clinics. Parents received written information about the study when attending for the second primary vaccination and were asked if they wished to participate when they returned for the third vaccination. The only exclusion criteria were those normally applicable to a child receiving primary immunisations.[1]

Oxford Vaccine Group, University Department of Paediatrics, John Radcliffe Hospital, Oxford OX3 9DU
Linda Diggle
senior research nurse

ICRF/NHS Centre for Statistics in Medicine, Institute of Health Sciences, University of Oxford, Oxford OX3 7LF
Jonathan Deeks
senior medical statistician

Correspondence to: L Diggle
linda.diggle@paediatrics.oxford.ac.uk

BMJ 2000;321:931–3

Reproduced with permission from BMJ Publishing Group Ltd.

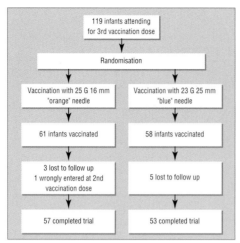

Flow chart describing randomisation sequence

We obtained ethical approval from the local ethics committee.

Interventions

Infants were allocated to receive their third primary immunisation with either the 25 gauge, 16 mm needle or the 23 gauge, 25 mm needle according to a computer generated blocked randomisation scheme stratified by practice. Allocations were concealed in sequentially numbered opaque envelopes opened once written parental consent was obtained. Practice nurses were instructed verbally, by demonstration and in writing, to use the technique of injecting into the anterolateral thigh, stretching the skin taut and inserting the needle at a 90° angle to the skin.[2] The right thigh was used, with the needle inserted into the skin up to the hub.

Outcomes

Parents recorded redness, swelling, and tenderness in a diary for three days after immunisation. The size of swelling and redness were measured with a plastic ruler, while the child's reaction to movement of the limb or to touch of the site was graded with a standard scale. We supplied parents with a prepaid envelope to return the diary, and we contacted parents by telephone if return was delayed.

At the start of the trial all practices were using the 0.5 ml mix of Pasteur-Merieux DPT/Hib vaccine. However, a change in national vaccine supply necessitated a switch to the 1.0 ml mix of Evans DPT and Wyeth Lederle Hib-Titer. Blocked randomisation ensured that the numbers receiving each vaccine were evenly distributed between the groups.

Statistical analysis

In order to detect clinically important relative differences of 25% in tenderness and 30% in redness

Baseline characteristics of 4 month old infants and rate of local reactions to immunisation over three days by needle used for vaccination. Values are numbers (percentages) of infants unless stated otherwise

Local reaction	Size of needle		Difference between longer and shorter needle	
	23 G, 25 mm (n=53)	25 G, 16 mm (n=57)	Relative risk (95% CI); P value	Test for trend
Baseline characteristics				
Mean (SD) weight (kg)*	6.7 (0.9)	6.8 (0.9)		
Age at vaccination (weeks):				
16-17	37 (70)	36 (63)		
18-19	11 (21)	16 (28)		
≥20	5 (9)	5 (9)		
Sex				
Male	34 (64)	30 (53)		
Female	19 (36)	27 (47)		
Site of injection:				
Left leg	13 (25)	12 (21)		
Right leg	40 (75)	45 (79)		
Vaccine type†:				
0.5 ml	8 (15)	8 (14)		
1.0 ml	45 (85)	49 (86)		
Local reactions				
Redness:				
At 6 hours	21 (40)	34 (60)	0.66 (0.45 to 0.99); P=0.04	P=0.007
At 1 day	15 (28)	36 (63)	0.45 (0.28 to 0.72); P=0.0002	P<0.0001
At 2 days	5 (9)	22 (39)	0.24 (0.10 to 0.60); P=0.0004	P=0.0004
At 3 days	2 (4)	16 (28)	0.13 (0.03 to 0.56); P=0.0006	P=0.001
Swelling:				
At 6 hours	12 (23)	33 (58)	0.39 (0.23 to 0.67); P=0.0002	P=0.0009
At 1 day	15 (28)	36 (63)	0.45 (0.28 to 0.72); P=0.0002	P=0.0001
At 2 days	10 (19)	29 (51)	0.37 (0.20 to 0.69); P=0.0005	P=0.0007
At 3 days	7 (13)	23 (40)	0.33 (0.15 to 0.70); P=0.001	P=0.002
Tenderness:				
At 6 hours	9 (17)	16 (28)	0.60 (0.29 to 1.25); P=0.17	P=0.4
At 1 day	4 (8)	8 (14)	0.54 (0.17 to 1.68); P=0.3	P=0.4
At 2 days	0	3 (5)	0 (not estimable); P=0.09	P=0.4
At 3 days	0	1 (2)	0 (not estimable); P=0.3	P=0.2
Any local reaction	33 (62)	48 (84)	0.74 (0.58 to 0.94); P=0.009	

*Weight missing for three infants.
†0.5 ml vaccine=Pasteur Merieux DPT/Hib. 1 ml vaccine=Evans DPT reconstituting Wyeth Lederle Hib-Titer.

Reproduced with permission from BMJ Publishing Group Ltd.

and swelling, we estimated that 250 infants should be recruited for the study to have 80% power of detecting differences at the 5% significance level. In January 2000, problems with vaccine supply necessitated the temporary nationwide replacement of the whole cell component of the combined DPT/Hib vaccine with acellular pertussis vaccine.[3] As this vaccine has a different local reactogenicity profile, we decided to stop the trial early.

We used χ^2 tests to compare the proportions of children with each local reaction at 6 hours and 1, 2, and 3 days after immunisation. We compared differences in the size of reaction using a χ^2 test for trend.

Results

Of the 119 children recruited to the study, 61 were randomised to the 16 mm needle group and 58 to the 25 mm needle group (see figure). Nine were not included in the analysis (four in the 16 mm needle group and five in the 25 mm group): diaries were not returned for eight, while the ninth was mistakenly included in the study at the second vaccination. Inclusion of this child did not materially affect the results. The two groups had similar baseline characteristics (see table).

Over half of the infants vaccinated with the 16 mm needle subsequently experienced redness and swelling (table). The rate of redness with the 25 mm needle was initially two thirds the rate with the 16 mm needle (relative risk 0.66 (95% confidence interval 0.45 to 0.99)), and, by the third day, this had decreased further to a seventh (relative risk 0.13 (0.03 to 0.56)). Similarly, rates of swelling after injection with the longer needle were initially around a third of those after use of the smaller needle (relative risk 0.39 (0.23 to 0.67)), and this difference was maintained for all three days. These differences were statistically significant. Tenderness was less frequent and, although the rates of tenderness were also lower with the longer needle throughout follow up, the differences were not significant (table).

Discussion

This study showed that both redness and swelling were significantly reduced when the 23 gauge, 25 mm, blue hub needle was used instead of the 25 gauge, 16 mm, orange hub needle to administer the third dose of diphtheria, pertussis, and tetanus and *Haemophilus influenzae* type b vaccines to infants. The differences suggest that, for every three to five infants vaccinated with the longer rather than the shorter needle, one case of redness and one of swelling would be prevented.

The needles compared in this study are those most commonly used in general practice.[4] As they differed in both length (16 v 25 mm) and bore (25 v 23 gauge), we cannot know which of these factors determined the observed differences in the rates of redness and swelling. However, previous studies comparing injections given at different depths (subcutaneous versus intramuscular) with the same gauge needle have shown similar differences in local reactions.[5] [6] We suggest that the length of the longer needle used in our

What is already known on this topic
Most infants experience local reactions to routine vaccinations
Previous local reactions have been cited by parents as a disincentive to further vaccinations
National guidelines on immunisation do not specify a preferred needle length

What this study adds
Local reactions are significantly reduced by use of the 23 gauge, 25 mm, blue hub needle rather than the 25 gauge, 16 mm, orange hub needle supplied by vaccine manufacturers

study ensured that the vaccine reached the thigh muscle in 4 month old infants.

Although our study was not blinded, parents were not told which needle was used to vaccinate their child. We believe that if knowledge of needle allocation introduced bias into the results, it would be less likely that such bias would be in the direction of the longer needle.

These findings are of clinical importance for those involved in administering infant immunisations. In the United Kingdom, where routine vaccines are currently supplied with the shorter needle, a change in the manufacturing process is now required. Any factor that can reduce the rates of adverse reactions in childhood vaccinations has the potential to improve parental acceptance of vaccines[7] and would be welcomed by practitioners.

We thank the parents and babies involved in the study, and the following practice nurses at Buckinghamshire surgeries for recruiting infants and administering immunisations: Lyn Hurry, Waddesdon; Lyn Murphy, Whitehill; Carol Gill, Aston Clinton; Judith Brown, Meadowcroft; Cesca Carter, Wendover; Nicky Oliver, Oakfield; Chris Mildred, Wing; Clare Stroud, Tring Road. We also thank Professor Richard Moxon and Drs Paul Heath, Jim Buttery, Jodie McVernon, Jenny MacLennan, and Karen Sleeman from the Oxford Vaccine Group for helpful advice and support and Dr Ann Mulhall for research supervision.

Contributors: LD conceived and planned the study, recruited and trained practice nurses, managed data collection, wrote the first draft of the paper, and is guarantor for the study. JD advised on design, produced the randomisation scheme, and undertook all analyses. Both authors had input into the final manuscript.

Funding: This study was funded by the Smith and Nephew Foundation through the award of a nursing research scholarship.

Competing interests: None declared.

1 Department of Health. *Immunisation against infectious diseases.* London: HMSO, 1996.
2 World Health Organisation. *Immunisation in practice. Module 8. During a session: giving immunisations.* Geneva: WHO, 1998. (www.who.int/vaccines-documents/DoxTrng/H4IIP.htm (accessed 3 October 2000).)
3 Department of Health. *Current vaccine issues: action update.* London: DoH, 1999. (Professional letter PL/CMO/99/5.)
4 Diggle L. A randomised controlled trial of different needle lengths on the incidence of local reactions when administering the combined injection of diphtheria/pertussis/tetanus (DPT) and Haemophilus influenzae type b (Hib) to infants at 4-months of age [dissertation]. London: Royal College of Nursing Institute, 1999.
5 Mark A, Carlsson R, Granstrom M. Subcutaneous versus intramuscular injection for booster DT vaccination of adolescents. *Vaccine* 1999;17:2067-72.
6 Scheifele DW, Bjornson G, Boraston S. Local adverse effects of meningococcal vaccine. *Can Med Assoc J* 1994;150:14-5.
7 Lieu T, Black S, Ray G, Martin K, Shinefield H, Weniger B. The hidden costs of infant vaccination. *Vaccine* 2000;19:33-41.

(Accepted 22 September 2000)

Reproduced with permission from BMJ Publishing Group Ltd.

Principles of critical appraisal — secondary research

Reviews of the scientific literature range from objective, quantitative information syntheses of the best research evidence, to highly subjective and selective summaries. The challenge for critically appraising secondary research is to decide where along this spectrum the review lies. This involves looking at the same three questions that we have already considered for primary research (individual studies):

▶ Question 1: What is the PICO of the study and is it close enough to your PICO?

▶ Question 2: How well was the study done?

▶ Question 3: What do the results mean and could they have been due to chance?

In this section, we will consider the principles involved in answering these questions and apply these principles to a systematic review of studies for an intervention question. See shaded sections with the logo:

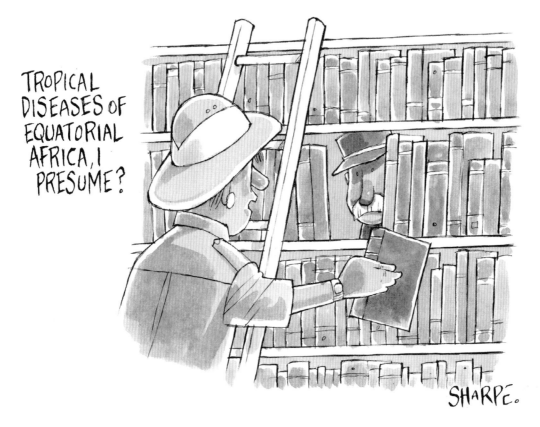

Critical appraisal of a systematic review of intervention studies

In this section, we will imagine that you have been investigating a topical question for older patients — whether corticosteroid injections into the knee joint improve the symptoms of osteoarthritis of the knee.

Reduction of symptoms of osteoarthritis of the knee

P *Population/problem* = older people (over 50 years of age) with osteoarthritis of the knee

I *Intervention* = corticosteroid injections into the knee joint

C *Comparator* = no injection

O *Outcome* = reduction in symptoms

Clinical question

In older people (> 50 years), do corticosteroid injections into the knee joint, compared with no injections, reduce the symptoms of osteoarthritis?

Search

A search in PubMed: ClinicalQueries using the terms:

corticosteroid AND knee* AND osteoarthrit*

... brings up a few review papers, of which the most recent and largest is a Cochrane review published in 2005. While you might wish to go straight to the Cochrane review, for this exercise, we want you to imagine that the only published review for this issue is one published in the BMJ in 2004:

Arroll F, Goodyear-Smith F (2004). Corticosteroid injections for osteoarthritis of the knee: meta-analysis. *British Medical Journal* 328:869–873.

This review is more concise than the Cochrane review and shows the main features we need to discuss. The full paper is included on pages 119–123.

Authors' conclusion

The authors of this paper concluded that: 'Evidence supports short-term (up to two weeks) improvement of symptoms after intra-articular corticosteroid injection for osteoarthritis of the knee.... But how reliable is this conclusion? In the following pages, we will use the principles of critical appraisal to find out.

Question 1: What is the PICO of the study and is it close enough to your PICO?

Once again, before you start appraising a systematic review, it is worthwhile spending a moment working out what question (PICO) the review addressed. As we saw for primary research, this helps to orient you to the paper and to decide if it provides useful information relevant to your PICO (see also the discussion below on whether the question is clearly stated).

> ### Is the PICO of the corticosteroid study close enough to your PICO?
>
>
>
> Looking at the corticosteroids review, the I and O of the PICO can be identified from the Abstract and Introduction to the paper, while a quick look at Table 2 shows the population for the included studies. Again, it is much the same as our PICO. Therefore, it certainly looks as though it is worth continuing.

Question 2: How well was the study done?

Like primary research, secondary research and syntheses of information (such as systematic reviews, clinical practice guidelines and decision tools) are prone to a variety of biases, such as:

▶ bias in the published studies that are chosen for inclusion in the review (selection bias), or in the choice of studies that are published in the first place (publication bias)

▶ bias in the level of importance attributed to the study results by the secondary researcher

▶ bias in the way that the results are summarised and presented.

In this section, we will describe how these problems can be minimised in secondary research using the corticosteroid paper as an example. Essentially, good-quality secondary research follows the first three steps that we have already been discussing for EBP. That is:

▶ formulate an answerable question   **Q**

▶ find the best evidence   **F**

▶ critically appraise the evidence   **A**

However, whereas we have been discussing how EBP can be used by practitioners to find information very quickly in order to guide decision making for a specific patient, a systematic review (or other type of secondary research) may take many months to complete and involves an extremely thorough search of the literature and analysis of the included studies.

The fourth step of secondary research is to 'synthesise' the results of the included studies and use them to formulate the conclusion of the research (**S**).

A comparison of the steps of EBP and the steps of secondary research (in this case for a systematic review) is shown in the table below.

Comparison of EBP and secondary research

Steps	EBP	Secondary research (eg a systematic review)	Critical appraisal issue
Q	Formulate a question (PICO)	Formulate a question (PICO)	Does the research ask a clearly focused question (PICO) and use it to direct the search and select articles for inclusion?
F	Find the best evidence	Find the best evidence	Did the search find all the best evidence?
A	Appraise the included studies	Appraise the included studies	Have the studies been critically appraised?
S	—	Synthesise the results (summary tables and plots)	Have the results been synthesised with appropriate summary tables and plots?
	Apply the results	—	See EBP Step 4: Apply the evidence
Comments	Time: < 2 minutes 1 practitioner 1–20 articles Can apply findings to *this* patient	Time: 6 months + Team of researchers Up to 2000 articles Cannot apply findings to *this* patient, but future patients may benefit from the summary of evidence	

Question — Did the research ask a clearly focused question?

Secondary research can be derailed because the researchers do not ask a focused question and instead start looking at a range of loosely connected articles in the hope that the right questions will eventually emerge. This approach may be appropriate when a researcher is conducting a scoping study of a new area, but it will not do if the aim of the research is to find out what works and what doesn't to aid specific health care decisions.

Therefore, the first thing to check is whether the main question being addressed is clearly stated. Ideally, it should be possible to identify all the PICO elements from the introduction and methods section of the paper. However, as a minimum, the intervention or exposure (such as a therapy or diagnostic test) and the outcome(s) should be expressed in terms of a simple relationship.

It is important for reviews to have a focused research question so that the question can be used to direct the search, as we have seen in EBP Step 2, and to set criteria for which articles to include for further assessment.

As well as criteria related to the PICO, researchers often use study type as the main criterion (for example, by only including RCTs). Excluded studies should also be recorded with reasons for the exclusions.

This helps to eliminate a major source of bias and subjectivity in secondary research, called 'selection bias'. Selection bias is similar to a primary researcher choosing which data to include in their results — obviously if only the 'best' data are included, the paper will be misleading.

> ### Steps in critical appraisal for secondary studies
>
> #### Question
> Does the research ask a clearly focused question (PICO) and use it to direct the search?
>
> #### Find
> Did the search find all the best evidence?
>
> #### Appraise
> Have the studies been critically appraised?
>
> #### Synthesise
> Have the results been synthesised with appropriate summary tables and plots?

Question — Did the corticosteroid reviewers ask a focused research question?

The corticosteroid review includes the following information on the objectives of the review and the selection of papers:

'Objectives: To determine the efficacy of intra-articular corticosteroid injections for osteoarthritis of the knee...'

See 'Abstract' (CS review p1).

'Efficacy' is also defined as 'improving the symptoms of osteoarthritis of the knee'.

See 'Introduction', last paragraph (CS review p1).

'Our selection criterion was randomised placebo controlled trials in which the efficacy of intra-articular corticosteroids for osteoarthritis of the knee, of any duration, could be assessed.'

See 'Methods' (CS review p1) and Fig 1 'Summary of search results' (CS review p2).

10 RCTs were included on this basis from 36 papers initially identified.

Find — Did the search find all the best evidence?

Search strategy

The first step in avoiding selection bias is using objective, systematic methods for finding all the high-quality papers that relate to the research question. Good-quality secondary research therefore includes a search protocol that clearly shows the methods used to search the literature. This should involve searching The Cochrane Library and the major electronic databases of published studies (such as PubMed [for MEDLINE] and EMBASE; see EBP Step 2: Track down the best evidence).

As not all studies are included in the databases and some may not be revealed by the keywords used, the search should also include some hand searching of relevant journals, conference proceedings and/or reference lists of articles found in the searches. Ideally, the review should include non-English as well as English language papers.

Overcoming publication bias

However careful researchers may be in finding all the *published* papers for a specific topic, much primary research will still be missed because of 'publication bias'. This occurs because authors and journal editors like to publish papers that show positive results but are more reluctant to publish those that show null or negative results. Indeed, researchers often do not even submit papers that do not support their hypothesis (ie show null or negative results).

However, to make sense of a body of evidence, null and negative results are just as important as positive ones. Therefore, good-quality secondary research needs to take account of unpublished studies as well as published ones. How this is done should be discussed in the methods section or protocol for the research and may include checking clinical trials registries (such as Current Controlled Trials, which is a meta-registry of controlled trials at http://www.controlled-trials.com); contacting experts working in the specific area of the research to ask if they know of any relevant unpublished research; and checking conference proceedings, the internet and other sources of unpublished literature.

Steps in critical appraisal for secondary studies

Question

Does the research ask a clearly focused question (PICO) and use it to direct the search?

Find

Did the search find all the best evidence?

Appraise

Have the studies been critically appraised?

Synthesise

Have the results been synthesised with appropriate summary tables and plots?

Find — Did the corticosteroid reviews find all the best evidence?

Search protocol

'We searched MEDLINE (1966 to 2003), and EMBASE (1980 to 2003)'

'The reference lists [of included studies] were scrutinised for relevant papers.'

'We searched the Cochrane controlled trials register'

How did the corticosteroid reviewers overcome publication bias?

'Authors of included studies were contacted for details of any further work.'

See 'Methods' (CS review p1).

Towards compulsory registration of clinical trials

In September 2004, the members of the International Committee of Medical Journal Editors, representing eleven prestigious medical journals, made a bold move to reduce publication bias. They announced that, for trials that started recruiting from 1 July 2005, they would only publish the results if the trial was registered on a publicly available registry before the enrolment of the first patient. The goal of this initiative is to foster a comprehensive, publicly available database of all clinical trials.

The World Health Organization (WHO) has also promoted the goal of a single worldwide standard for the information that trial authors must disclose, and governments around the world have started to introduce legislation for mandatory disclosure of all trials.

See further information at:

http://www.who.int/mediacentre/news/releases/2006/pr25/en/index.html

http://www.controlled-trials.com/

Reference:

De Angelis C, Drazen JM, Frizelle FA, Haug C, et al (2004). Clinical trial registration: a statement from the International Committee of Medical Journal Editors. *Annals of Internal Medicine* 141:477–478.

Appraise — Have the studies been critically appraised?

Even if the searching has been done very well, the validity of the results and conclusions of the review will depend on the quality of the individual included studies.

Therefore, a good-quality secondary research paper or report should include a critical appraisal for each of the studies showing the quality of the studies in terms of the RAMMbo checklist described in this workbook on page 77 (or similar).

As critical assessment can be subjective, ideally, each study should be appraised by two assessors working independently. Any points of disagreement should be discussed and a consensus reached.

If any studies are excluded from further analysis based on the critical appraisal, they should be listed with the other excluded studies with the reasons stated. A good appraisal will do two things:

▶ say what the minimum required study quality was for inclusion

▶ give a clear picture of the quality and limitations of the included studies.

Appraise — How did the corticosteroid reviewers appraise the studies?

'The two authors independently assessed the methodological quality using the Jadad scoring system. Consensus was reached through discussion.'

See 'Methods' (CS review p1) and Table 1 'Jadad quality scores...' (CS review p2).

Steps in critical appraisal for secondary studies

Question

Does the research ask a clearly focused question (PICO) and use it to direct the search?

Find

Did the search find all the best evidence?

Appraise

Have the studies been critically appraised?

Synthesise

Have the results been synthesised with appropriate summary tables and plots?

Synthesise — Have the results been synthesised with appropriate summary tables and plots?

The final quality issue for secondary research is how well the results have been extracted and summarised. As for the appraisal step, to reduce any bias of the reviewers, it is a good idea if the data is extracted from the included studies by two assessors working independently. The two assessors can then compare notes and resolve any discrepancies.

The most appropriate way to present the results will depend on the purpose of the secondary research (eg for a systematic review and meta-analysis, clinical practice guidelines or decision tool). There should at least be a succinct summary of the included studies (usually in a table) showing the types of studies, interventions or exposures tested, numbers of subjects, the results of the critical appraisal and the results (including 95% confidence intervals) of each separate study. Graphic presentations such as 'forest plots', are also helpful (see below) and, for a meta-analysis, the summary measure, confidence intervals and heterogeneity should also be included.

If different results have been obtained in the individual studies, it will be difficult to draw firm conclusions from the review. The tables and plots should therefore indicate whether the results were similar from study to study, or whether there were any major differences (heterogeneity).

Heterogeneity suggests that there must have been other factors in the studies to account for the different results, and the authors of the review should include a discussion of what these might have been. They may be either the PICO elements (differences in population, interventions, comparators and outcome measures) or the methodological quality of the studies. See below for some further discussion of heterogeneity.

Steps in critical appraisal for secondary studies

Question

Does the research ask a clearly focused question (PICO) and use it to direct the search?

Find

Did the search find all the best evidence?

Appraise

Have the studies been critically appraised?

Synthesise

Have the results been synthesised with appropriate summary tables and plots?

Synthesise — Did the corticosteroid reviewers synthesise the results using appropriate summary tables and plots?

'Table 2 Details of included studies with outcomes on improvement in osteoarthritis of the knee '

This table shows a summary of the 10 included studies with information about the patients and type of osteoarthritis suffered, intervention and control groups, and outcomes.

See 'Results', Table 2 (CS review p3).

Figures 2, 3 and 4 show forest plots for 3 improvements in osteoarthritis symptoms and include statistical analysis of heterogeneity.

See 'Results', Figs 2–4 (CS review p4).

Question 3: What do the results mean?

Secondary research, such as a systematic review, provides a summary of the data from the results of a number of individual studies.

If the results of the individual studies are similar, a statistical method (called meta-analysis) can be used to combine the results from the individual studies and an overall summary estimate is calculated.

The meta-analysis gives weighted values to each of the individual studies according to their size. The individual results of the studies need to be expressed in a standard way, such as relative risk, odds ratio or mean difference between the groups. The results of the analysis are traditionally displayed in a figure, like the one below, called a **forest plot**.

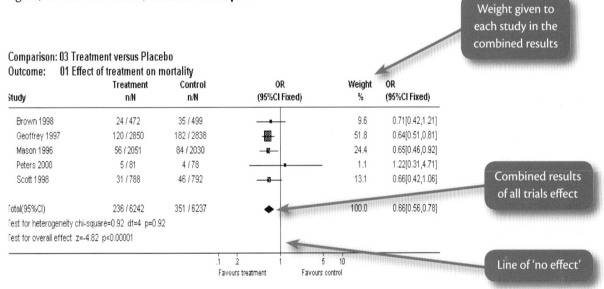

Note: See the 'Glossary' in Part 4 of this workbook for a definition of odds ratio.

The forest plot depicted above represents a meta-analysis of five trials that assessed the effects of a hypothetical treatment on mortality. Individual studies are represented by a black square and a horizontal line, which correspond to the point estimate and 95% CI of the odds ratio respectively (see the previous section on primary research for further explanation of what these terms mean).

The size (area) of the black square reflects the weight of the study in the meta-analysis. The solid vertical line corresponds to 'no effect' of treatment—that is, an odds ratio of 1.0. When the confidence interval includes 1, it indicates that the result is not significant at conventional levels ($P > 0.05$).

The diamond at the bottom represents the combined or pooled odds ratio of all five trials with its 95% CI. In this case, it shows that the treatment reduces mortality by 34% (OR 0.66, 95% CI 0.56 to 0.78). Notice that the diamond does not overlap the 'no effect' line (the confidence interval doesn't include 1), so we can conclude that the pooled OR is statistically significant. The test for overall effect also indicates statistical significance ($P < 0.0001$).

Exploring heterogeneity

Heterogeneity can be assessed using the 'eyeball' test or more formally with statistical tests, such as I^2 and the Cochran chi-square (Q) test. With the 'eyeball' test, you look for overlap of the confidence intervals of the trials with the summary estimate. The amount of heterogeneity is calculated as the I^2 value (0 if none; near 1 if a lot) and the statistical significance of this value can be assessed using the Cochran Q test.

▶ If Cochran Q is statistically significant, there is definite heterogeneity.

▶ If Cochran Q is not statistically significant but the ratio of Cochran Q and the degrees of freedom (Q/df) is greater than 1, there is possible heterogeneity.

▶ If Cochran Q is not statistically significant and Q/df is less then 1, then heterogeneity is very unlikely.

In the example above, Q/df is less then 1 (0.92/4= 0.23) and the P-value is not significant (0.92) indicating no heterogeneity.

Note: The level of significance for Cochran Q is often set at 0.1 due to the low power of the test to detect heterogeneity.

To make decisions about the worth of a treatment, good information about adverse effects or treatment is important, but this is often lacking in both individual trials and systematic reviews.

What do the results of the corticosteroid review mean?

The corticosteroid paper provides three forest plots.

Figure 2: Improvements up to two weeks after steroid injection in knee
Six studies included this outcome. Only three of the individual studies are statistically significant and one of these has a very large CI. However, the summary estimate shows RR = 1.66 (95% CI 1.37 to 2.01), which does not cross 1 (the ratio for 'no effect') and hence is a statistically significant improvement.

▸ Heterogeneity score (Cochran Q): P = 0.12 (not significant); df = 5; Q/df = 0.024 (< 1)

▸ This indicates that heterogeneity is unlikely.

▸ Around 45% of the patients improved with placebo (the control event rate). The number needed to treat (NNT) to obtain one improvement based on the summary estimate was 3.5.

Figure 3: Improvements at 16–24 weeks after high-dose steroid injection in knee for two high-quality studies

Two high-quality studies included this outcome. Neither of the studies is statistically significant.

▸ However, the summary estimate shows RR = 2.09 (95% CI 1.20 to 3.65), which is a statistically significant improvement

▸ Heterogeneity score (Cochran Q): P = 0.83 (not significant); df = 1; Q/df = 0.83 (< 1)

▸ This indicates that heterogeneity is unlikely.

▸ Around 21% of the patients improved with placebo (control event rate); NNT = 4.4.

Figure 4: Levels of pain recorded for up to two weeks after steroid injection
Five studies showed this outcome. The summary estimate shows RR = −16.47 (95%CI −22.92 to −10.03), which is a statistically significant reduction in pain.

Summary of the critical appraisal of the corticosteroid review

Internal validity

Question

The corticosteroid review is a systematic review based on a clear clinical question and the PICO is similar to ours.

Find

The inclusion criteria and search methods are stated in the methods section. Inclusion criteria were based on the clinical question.

A comprehensive search of the literature was conducted, including MEDLINE (PubMed) and EMBASE. The researchers contacted the authors of included papers directly and checked the reference lists for further relevant papers. They also searched the Cochrane controlled trial register for unpublished clinical trials.

36 studies were retrieved, of which 10 were included. The excluded studies are not listed with individual reasons for exclusions.

Appraise

Only RCTs were considered. The studies were critically appraised using the Jadad quality scores and the scores are shown in the paper.

Synthesise

The paper includes a clear summary table of the included studies, with forest plots and heterogeneity analysis for three outcome measures.

Results

The results show statistically significant improvement in symptoms, including reduction in pain, for up to 2 weeks after corticosteroid injections at a range of doses. Two studies also showed statistically significant improvement in symptoms at 16–24 weeks after injection of a higher dose. Heterogeneity analysis in each case showed that heterogeneity was unlikely.

There was no mention of side-effects in the paper, which means we may have to look elsewhere for this. For example, how common were local reactions or infection?

Overall conclusion

The study is a good-quality systematic review that shows a statistically significant reduction in symptoms of osteoarthritis after corticosteroid injections at various doses. Further work is needed on the relationship between the duration of symptom relief and dose.

Primary care

Corticosteroid injections for osteoarthritis of the knee: meta-analysis

Bruce Arroll, Felicity Goodyear-Smith

Abstract

Objectives To determine the efficacy of intra-articular corticosteroid injections for osteoarthritis of the knee and to identify numbers needed to treat.

Data sources Cochrane controlled trials register, Medline (1966 to 2003), Embase (1980 to 2003), hand searches, and contact with authors.

Inclusion criteria Randomised controlled trial in which the efficacy of intra-articular corticosteroid injections for osteoarthritis of the knee could be ascertained.

Results In high quality studies, the pooled relative risk for improvement in symptoms of osteoarthritis of the knee at 16-24 weeks after intra-articular corticosteroid injections was 2.09 (95% confidence interval 1.2 to 3.7) and the number needed to treat was 4.4. The pooled relative risk for improvement up to two weeks after injections was 1.66 (1.37 to 2.0). The numbers needed to treat to get one improvement in the statistically significant studies was 1.3 to 3.5 patients.

Conclusion Evidence supports short term (up to two weeks) improvement in symptoms of osteoarthritis of the knee after intra-articular corticosteroid injection. Significant improvement was also shown in the only methodologically sound studies addressing longer term response (16-24 weeks). A dose equivalent to 50 mg of prednisone may be needed to show benefit at 16-24 weeks.

Introduction

Knee pain is relatively common. Around a quarter of people aged 55 years or more in the United Kingdom and the Netherlands have persistent pain, and one in six will consult their general practitioner.[1] Osteoarthritis is the single most common cause of disability in older adults, with 10% of patients aged 55 or more having painful disabling osteoarthritis of the knee, a quarter of whom are severely disabled.[1] With no cure (excluding joint replacement), treatment is directed at pain relief and improvement or maintenance of function.

Intra-articular injection of steroid is a common treatment for osteoarthritis of the knee. Clinical evidence suggests that benefit is short lived, usually one to four weeks.[2] The short term effect of steroids shown by controlled trials and clinical experience vary, however, with some patients seen by rheumatologists achieving a significant and sustained response beyond a few weeks. This may be explained by only one injection usually being given in clinical trials and at a lower dose (20 mg) than the 40 mg triamcinolone recommended by the American College of Rheumatologists.[3] Pain scores may also be an insensitive outcome measure.

Concern has been expressed that long term treatment could promote joint destruction and tissue atrophy.[2] Studies of cartilage damage, however, tend to suggest that changes are more likely due to the underlying disease than the steroid injection.[4]

Three papers have reviewed the general management of osteoarthritis of the knee, one specifically on corticosteroid injections, but no meta-analysis has been undertaken.[1 4-6] We therefore performed a meta-analysis to determine whether intra-articular injections of corticosteroid are more efficacious than placebo in improving the symptoms of osteoarthritis of the knee.

Methods

We searched the Cochrane controlled trials register, Medline (1966 to 2003), and Embase (1980 to 2003) using the MeSH terms triamcinolone; prednisolone; prednisone; hydrocortisone; adrenal cortex hormones; osteoarthritis; knee; injections, intra-articular; and randomized controlled trial, and the non-MeSH terms injections; randomised controlled trial; and corticosteroid and steroid. Authors of included studies were contacted for details of any further work. The reference lists were scrutinised for relevant papers.

Our selection criterion was randomised placebo controlled trials in which the efficacy of intra-articular corticosteroids for osteoarthritis of the knee, of any duration, could be assessed. We considered improvement as the most important patient oriented outcome. Terms used to determine the discrete outcomes were distinct improvement, subjective improvement, decreased pain, overall improvement, clinically relevant outcomes, and response to the osteoarthritis research scale.[7-12] Numbers needed to treat were calculated from dichotomous outcomes.[13]

The two authors independently assessed the methodological quality using the Jadad scoring system.[14] Consensus was reached through discussion. Data extraction was similarly achieved. Data were analysed with Review Manager 4.1 (Update Software, Oxford). We calculated the relative risk and number needed to treat for improvement. An a priori subgroup analysis was conducted for study quality, dose of drug, duration of effect, specialty of injector, and condition of the knee. The dose equivalents were obtained from elsewhere.[15] The conduct of this review was undertaken according to the QUOROM statement.[16]

Results

Ten trials met the inclusion criteria (fig 1).[2 7-12 17-19] An additional paper examined intra-articular corticosteroid injections postoperatively, but we did not consider this paper in the review.[20] Table 1 shows the quality scores of the included studies, and table 2 summarises details of the studies and improvements attained.

Six studies provided data on improvement of symptoms of osteoarthritis of the knee after intra-articular corticosteroid injections (fig 2). These showed a significant improvement (rela-

Reproduced with permission from BMJ Publishing Group Ltd.

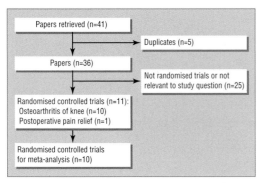

Fig 1 Summary of search results

tive risk 1.66, 95% confidence interval 1.37 to 2.01). For the statistically significant studies the number needed to treat to obtain one improvement was between 1.3 and 3.5. No important harms were reported other than transient redness and discomfort. Only one study investigated potential loss of joint space and found no difference between corticosteroid and placebo up to two years.[2]

Neither of the two high quality studies were statistically significant for improvement at 16 to 24 weeks, but the pooled result gave a relative risk of 2.09 (1.20 to 3.65) with a number needed to treat of 4.4 based on this result (fig 3). Significant heterogeneity was found when the one low quality study was included. The result was non-significant by random effects analysis. Figure 4 shows the results of pooling the 100 mm visual analogue scale for five studies. When standard deviations were not reported, we assigned a value of 30, as this was the highest reported value and was taken as a conservative estimate. This result is statistically significant. We found no results for pain 16 weeks after injection. A funnel plot of the six studies suggested that there was an absence of small studies with small effects (fig 5). The smallest study had 12 patients and the largest 71.

A similar result was found for improvement up to two weeks for the high dose studies. The effect at 16 to 24 weeks for these studies was the same as the two high quality studies. It was not possible to make a definitive analysis of the clinical conditions of the knee. The patients seemed to have mainly mild to moderate osteoarthritis. The dose equivalent to prednisone varied from 6.25 mg to 80 mg.

Discussion

Intra-articular injections of corticosteroid improve symptoms of osteoarthritis of the knee. Effects were beneficial up to two weeks

and at 16 to 24 weeks. This is the first meta-analysis on this topic and the first review to show benefits of such injections in improvement of symptoms, which may extend beyond 16 weeks. We also report clinically significant numbers needed to treat, ranging between 1.3 and 3.5 patients. The one study that investigated potential loss of joint space found no difference between corticosteroid and placebo up to two years.[2] This study also used a higher dose of triamcinolone (40 mg) than most of the other studies (20 mg) and gave repeated injections (every three months for two years).

Responses to intra-articular corticosteroids injections vary between the clinical experience of rheumatologists, where some patients have a significant and sustained response, to the short term benefit shown by randomised controlled trials.[4] Trials tend to use one injection only and at lower doses than the recommended 20 mg triamcinolone.[3] Subjective pain scales may also be an insensitive outcome measure in this condition.[4]

One limitation of our review is possible publication bias, in that by missing unpublished trials or those that showed negative effects we may have overestimated the benefits of corticosteroid injections. We believe, however, that our comprehensive, systematic search strategy enabled us to identify most research in this discipline. Another limitation of our study was the small size of the included studies.

Unlike other reviews we report improvement in symptoms, as we believe this is a more important patient oriented outcome than increases in range of movement or pain reduction.[21] Only the review by Pendleton and coworkers attempted to pool the results of papers, but they did not perform a meta-analysis, rather they reported the number of studies that showed benefits compared with those that did not and a median effect size.[5] Apart from the fact that other reviewers did not pool their data, we had the benefit of access to an article that was in press.[12] When this was added to the other two studies, the pooled result was statistically significant for the two high quality studies.[12] Larger studies are needed to confirm these findings.

The dose of corticosteroid required to improve symptoms is not clear from our review. The equivalent dose of prednisone varied from 6.25 mg to 80 mg.[12 19] A dose of 20 mg triamcinolone (equivalent to 25 mg of prednisone) seems to be efficacious for pain control at two weeks. Only one study used 40 mg triamcinolone, and this found a benefit at 24 months for night pain and stiffness on one scale but not on another.[2] This study also gave repeated injections and monitored loss of joint space (reporting no difference). The three studies that reported improvement at 16 weeks used different cortisones. The two

Table 1 Jadad quality scores for 10 studies of intra-articular corticosteroid injections for osteoarthritis of the knee

Study	1	2	3	4	5	6	7	8	9	10	11	Jadad score[14]
Cederlöf 1966[7]	+	+	?	?	+	?	+	+	+	+	−	3
Dieppe 1980[8]	+	+	?	+	?	−	+	+	+	+	+	3
Friedman 1980[9]	+	+	?	+	+	+	+	+	+	+	−	5
Gaffney 1995[10]	+	+	?	+	−	−	+	+	−	+	+	3
Jones 1996[17]	+	+	?	+	+	−	+	−	−	+	+	3
Miller 1958[18]	+	+	?	+	−	?	+	+	−	+	−	2
Ravaud 1999[11]	+	+	?	+	+	+	+	+	+	+	+	5
Raynauld 2003[2]	+	+	?	+	−	−	+	+	+	+	+	3
Smith 2003[12]	+	+	?	−	+	+	+	+	+	+	+	5
Wright 1960[19]	+	+	?	+	+	+	?	+	−	+	−	5

Numbers 1-11 follow Pedro format (www.cchs.usyd.edu.au/pedro/); Jadad score is calculated from different set of criteria[14]: 1=eligibility criteria specified; 2=patients randomised to groups; 3=concealment of allocation; 4=groups similar at baseline; 5=patients blinded; 6=practitioners administering intervention blinded; 7=assessors blinded; 8=measurements of key outcomes obtained from >85% of patients; 9=intention to treat analysis; 10=statistical comparisons between groups; 11=point measures and measures of variability provided.
+Criterion clearly satisfied.
−Criterion not clearly satisfied.
?Unclear whether criterion was satisfied.

Reproduced with permission from BMJ Publishing Group Ltd.

Table 2 Details of included studies with outcomes on improvement in osteoarthritis of knee

Study, location	Condition	Details of patients	Injectors; nature of injection	Outcome	Jadad score
Cederlöf 1966,[7] Sweden	History of aching after exertion, not trauma related and positive radiograph but no noticeable cartilage destruction	≥40 years; no details on sex or duration of osteoarthritis	Surgeons; aspiration and intra-articular steroid injection (Meticortelone 2 ml) compared with placebo (saline); prednisone equivalent 50 mg	No significant difference between groups at 1, 3, and 8 weeks. Results reported as distinct improvement. At one week, 18/26 in experimental group, 14/25 in control group; eight weeks, 17/26 in experimental group, 19/25 in control group had continued improvement compared with baseline	3/5
Dieppe 1980,[8] United Kingdom	Bilateral symptomatic osteoarthritis of knees	Mean 65 years; eight females, four males; most had grade 2-4 radiographic changes. Duration of osteoarthritis 7.5 years	Rheumatologist; aspiration and intra-articular steroid injection (triamcinolone hexacetonide 20 mg) compared with placebo (saline); prednisone equivalent 25 mg	Small, transient reduction in pain and tenderness compared with placebo. At one week, subjective improvement in 10/12 in experimental group, 1/12 in control group. Visual analogue scale at one week: mean 36 (SD 29) in experimental group, 70 (30) in control group	3/5
Friedman 1980,[9] United States	Mild to moderate changes on radiograph	42-75 years; mean duration of osteoarthritis 24 months for corticosteroid group and 36 months for placebo group	Rheumatologist; aspiration and intra-articular steroid injection (triamcinolone hexacetonide 20 mg) compared with placebo (saline); prednisone equivalent 25 mg	Steroid provided short term pain relief; at one week but not at 4, 6, 8 weeks. At one week described as decreased pain; 15/17 in experimental group, 12/17 in control group	5/5
Gaffney 1995,[10] United Kingdom	38% synovial fluid and knee pain for six months	Mean 67 years; 60 females, 24 males. Mean duration 6.7 years for corticosteroid group and 7.1 years for placebo group	Rheumatologist; aspiration and intra-articular steroid injection (triamcinolone hexacetonide 20 mg) compared with placebo (saline); prednisone equivalent 25 mg	Steroid provided short term pain relief. Benefit at one week but not at six weeks. At one week overall improvement; 33/42 in experimental group, 21/42 in control group. Visual analogue scale: mean 21.7 (SD 20.7) in experimental group, 43.1 (28.7) in control group	3/5
Jones 1996,[17] United Kingdom	Clinical and radiological osteoarthritis of knee	Mean 71 years; 23 males, 37 females. No details on duration of osteoarthritis	Rheumatologist; aspiration and intra-articular steroid injection (methylprednisolone 40 mg) compared with placebo (saline); prednisone equivalent 40 mg	Steroid provided short term pain relief. Responders at eight weeks: 28/30 in experimental group, 9/30 in control group	3/5
Miller 1958,[18] Scotland	Primary osteoarthritis	No details on age, sex, or duration of osteoarthritis	Unclear who injected; intra-articular steroid injection (hydrocortisone 50 mg) compared with lactic acid; local anaesthetic; saline; and mock injection. Injections given five times at two week intervals; prednisone equivalent 12.5 mg	Steroid did not provide improvement better than placebo at six weeks or six months follow up after completion of treatment. Term used was "improved." At six months: 4/34 in experimental group, 2/34 in control group; at 16 weeks 6/37 in experimental group, 8/36 in control group	2/5
Ravaud 1999,[11] France	Most had knee effusion; all had osteophytes and minimal joint space narrowing	Mean 63-67 years; 66 females, two males. No details on duration of osteoarthritis	Rheumatologist; intra-articular steroid injection (cortivazol 1.5 ml) with or without joint lavage compared with placebo (saline); prednisone equivalent 37.5 mg	Steroid provided short term pain relief up to four weeks but no effect at 24 weeks. At one week clinically relevant improvement in pain, 16/25 in experimental group and 7/28 in control group. At 24 weeks: 12/25 in experimental group and 6/28 in control group. Visual analogue scale at one week: (n=24) mean 23.7 (SD 26.2) in experimental group, (n=21) 45.7 (26.6) in control group	5/5
Raynauld 2003,[2] Canada	Kellgren and Lawrence grade 2 or 3	63 years; 67.5% female. Mean duration of osteoarthritis 9.8 years for corticosteroid group and 8.7 years for placebo group	Rheumatologist; intra-articular steroid injection (triamcinolone 40 mg) and placebo (saline) every three months for two years; prednisone equivalent 50 mg	Area under curve showed benefit for night pain and stiffness: 34 in each of experimental and control groups. At one year patient visual analogue scale: 34.32 (SD 20.9) in experimental group, 31.1 (21.1) in control group	3/5
Smith 2003,[12] Australia	Radiograph grade 2 or 3	Mean 66-67 years; 44 males, 27 females	Orthopaedic surgeon and rheumatologist; intra-articular steroid injection (methylprednisolone acetate 120 mg) after joint lavage compared with placebo; prednisone equivalent 80 mg	Steroid better than placebo only at four week follow up but not at 8, 12, or 24 weeks. Osteoarthritis Research Society response occurred: at two weeks 25/38 in experimental group, 15/33 in control group; at 24 weeks 16/38 in experimental group, 7/33 in control group. Visual analogue scale at two weeks: mean 20.8 (SD 30) in experimental group, 24.7 (30) in control group	5/5
Wright 1960,[19] United Kingdom	Denominator knees not pooled	No details on personal characteristics or duration of osteoarthritis	Internal medicine specialist; intra-articular steroid injections (hydrocortisone acetate 25 mg and hydrocortisone tertiary-butylacetate 25 mg) compared with placebo (injection vehicle). Four injections given at two weekly intervals; prednisone equivalent 6.25 mg	Both steroids provided transient pain relief at two weeks (25 patients, 38 knees)	5/5

Reproduced with permission from BMJ Publishing Group Ltd.

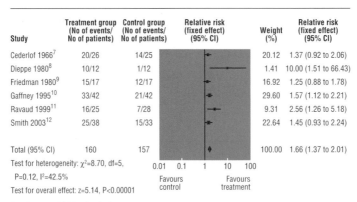

Fig 2 Improvements up to two weeks after steroid injection in knee

studies using high doses showed a statistically significant difference suggesting that higher dose steroids may give a longer benefit.[2] [12] It is not clear to whom the results of this study would apply.[11] [12] All the studies were done in hospital settings.

One study found that predicting benefit was not possible.[17] In contrast to another study, those who had synovial fluid aspirated had a better response.[10] This only occurred in the intervention group, ruling out that aspiration was associated with accurate placement of the needle. Another explanation is that the presence of knee effusion is correlated with the presence of synovitis and that intra-articular steroids my be effective against the inflammation.[4] One study recommended joint lavage combined with steroid injection if a knee effusion persisted after one or two steroid injections eight to 10 days apart.[4] Joint lavage was either efficacious (at two weeks) or nearly efficacious (efficacious when controlled for severity from radiographic evidence at 24 weeks) for more than 16 weeks.[11] [12]

Evidence supports short term (up to two weeks) improvement of symptoms from intra-articular corticosteroid injection for osteoarthritis of the knee, and the only methodologically-sound studies addressing longer term response (16-24 weeks) also show significant improvement. Doses of 50 mg equivalent of prednisone may be needed to obtain benefits at 16 to 24 weeks. Corticosteroid injection in addition to lavage needs further investigation. Currently no evidence supports the promotion of disease progression by steroid injections. Repeat injections seem to be safe over two years but needs confirmation from other studies.

Contributors: BA and FG-S were involved in extracting the data, appraising the article, and writing the paper. BA did the mathematical pooling; he will act as guarantor for the paper. The guarantor accepts full responsibility for the conduct of the study, had access to the data, and controlled the decision to publish.

Funding: This study was funded by the New Zealand Accident Rehabilitation and Compensation Insurance Corporation. Their role was limited to commissioning the work.

Competing interests: None declared.

Ethical approval: Not required.

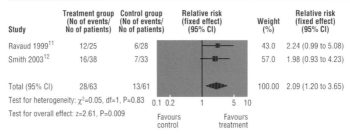

Fig 3 Improvements at 16-24 weeks after high dose steroid injection in knee for two high quality studies

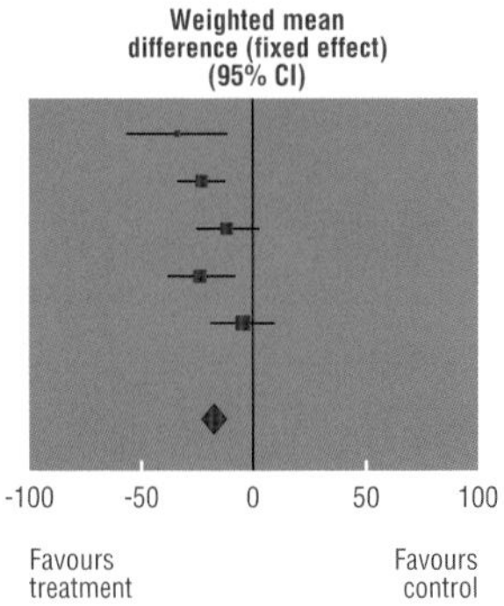

Fig 4 Visual analogue scale for pain up to two weeks after steroid injection in knee

Reproduced with permission from BMJ Publishing Group Ltd.

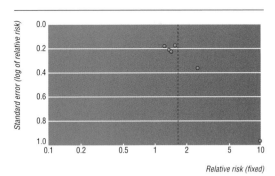

Fig 5 Funnel plot for corticosteroids compared with placebo

1 Peat G, McCarney R, Croft P. Knee pain and osteoarthritis in older adults: a review of community burden and current use of primary health care. *Ann Rheum Dis* 2001;60:91-7.

2 Raynauld J, Buckland-Wright C, Ward R, Choquette D, Haraoui B, Martel-Pelletier J, et al. Safety and efficacy of long-term intraarticular steroid injections in osteoarthritis of the knee. *Arth Rheum* 2003;48:370-7.

What is already known on this topic

Intra-articular corticosteroids provide short term (two weeks) relief of symptoms of osteoarthritis of the knee

Concerns are that multiple injections may damage articular cartilage

What this study adds

Intra-articular corticosteroids are probably effective in improving symptoms of osteoarthritis of the knee for 16 to 24 weeks

The number needed to treat is 4.4

Higher doses of cortisone (equivalent to 50 mg prednisone) may be more effective than lower doses, especially after 16 or more weeks

3 American College of Rheumatology subcommittee on osteoarthritis guidelines. Recommendations for the medical management of osteoarthritis of the hip and knee. *Arth Rheum* 2000;43:1905-15.

4 Ayral X. Injections in the treatment of osteoarthritis. *Best Pract Res Clin Rehumatol* 2001;15:609-26.

5 Pendleton A, Arden N, Dougados M, Doherty M, Bannwarth B, Bijlsma JW, et al. EULAR recommendations for the management of knee osteoarthritis: report of a task force of the Standing Committee for International Clinical Studies Including Therapeutic Trials (ESCISIT). *Ann Rheum Dis* 2000;59:936-44.

6 Mazieres B, Masquelier AM, Capron MH. A French controlled multicenter study of intraarticular orgotein versus intraarticular corticosteroids in the treatment of knee osteoarthritis: a one-year follow up. *J Rheumatol Suppl* 1991;27:134-7.

7 Cederlof S, Jonson G. Intraarticular prednisolone injection for osteoarthritis of the knee. A double blind test with placebo. *Acta Chir Scand* 1966;132:532-7.

8 Dieppe PA, Sathapatayavongs B, Jones HE, Bacon PA, Ring EF. Intra-articular steroids in osteoarthritis. *Rheumatol Rehabil* 1980;19:212-7.

9 Friedman DM, Moore ME. The efficacy of intraarticular steroids in osteoarthritis: a double-blind study. *J Rheumatol* 1980;7:850-6.

10 Gaffney K, Ledingham J, Perry JD. Intra-articular triamcinolone hexacetonide in knee osteoarthritis: factors influencing the clinical response. *Ann Rheum Dis* 1995;54:379-81.

11 Ravaud P, Moulinier L, Giraudeau B, Ayral X, Guerin C, Noel E, et al. Effects of joint lavage and steroid injection in patients with osteoarthritis of the knee: results of a multicenter, randomized, controlled trial. *Arth Rheum* 1999;42:475-82.

12 Smith MD, Wetherall M, Darby T, Esterman A, Slavotinek J, Robert-Thomson P, et al. A randomized placebo-controlled trial of arthroscopic lavage versus lavage plus intra-articular corticosteroids in the management of symptomatic osteoarthritis of the knee. *Rheumatol* 2003;42:1477-85.

13 Guyatt G, Juniper EF, Walter SD, Griffith LE, Goldstein RS. Interpreting treatment effects in randomised trials. *BMJ* 1998;316:690-3.

14 Jadad AR, Moore RA, Carroll D, Jenkinson C, Reynolds JM, Gavaghan DJ, et al. Assessing the quality of reports on randomised clinical trials: is blinding necessary? *Control Clin Trials* 1996;17:1-12.

15 Lane NE, Lukert B. The science and therapy of glucocorticoid-induced bone loss. *Endocrinol Metab Clin North Am* 1998;27:465-83.

16 Moher D, Cook D, Eastwood S, Olkin I, Rennie D, Stroup DF. Improving the quality of reports of meta-analyses of randomized controlled trials: the QUOROM statement. Quality of reporting of meta-analyses. *Lancet* 1999;354:1896-900.

17 Jones A, Doherty M. Intra-articular corticosteroids are effective in osteoarthritis but there are no clinical predictors of response. *Ann Rheum Dis* 1996;55:829-32.

18 Miller J, White J, Norton T. The value of intra-articular injections in osteoarthritis of the knee. *J Bone Joint Surg* 1958;4013:636-43.

19 Wright V, Chandler G, Morison R, Hartfall S. Intra-articular therapy in osteoarthritis. Comparison of hydrocortisone acetate and hydrocortisone teriary-butylacetate. *Ann Rheum Dis* 1960;19:257-61.

20 Wang JJ, Ho ST, Lee SC, Tang JJ, Liaw WJ. Intraarticular triamcinolone acetonide for pain control after arthroscopic knee surgery. *Anesth Analgesia* 1998;87:1113-6.

21 Liang MH, Lew RA, Stucki G, Fortin PR, Daltroy L. Measuring clinically important changes with patient-oriented questionnaires. *Med Care* 2002;40:II45-51.

(Accepted 21 January 2004)

doi 10.1136/bmj.38039.573970.7C

Department of General Practice and Primary Health Care, School of Population Health University of Auckland, Private Bag 92019 Auckland
Bruce Arroll *associate professor*
Felicity Goodyear-Smith *senior lecturer*

Correspondence to: B Arroll b.arroll@auckland.ac.nz

Reproduced with permission from BMJ Publishing Group Ltd.

Rapid critical appraisal of your own secondary research study for an intervention question

Now you can critically appraise the secondary research studies that you found during your earlier search session.

If you prefer, you can appraise the article on metoclopramide for acute migraine that is included at the end of this section.

For your chosen article, work through the critical appraisal sheet on the next few pages and then:

(a) decide whether the internal validity of the study is sufficient to allow firm conclusions (all studies have some flaws; but are these flaws bad enough to discard the study?)

(b) if the study is sufficiently valid, look at and interpret the results — what is the relevance or size of the effects of the intervention?

Rapid critical appraisal of a systematic review

Step 1: What question did the study ask?

Population/problem: ....

Intervention: ....

Comparison: ....

Outcome(s): ....

Step 2: How well was the study done? (internal validity)

Question — Does the systematic review address a focused question (PICO)?	
What is best?	**Where do I find the information?**
The main question being addressed should be clearly stated. The exposure, such as a therapy or diagnostic test, and the outcome(s) of interest will often be expressed in terms of a simple relationship.	The **Title**, **Abstract** or **final paragraph** of the **Introduction** should clearly state the question. If you still cannot ascertain what the focused question is after reading these sections, search for another paper!

This paper: Yes ☐   No ☐   Unclear ☐   Comment: ....

... and use it to direct the search and select articles for inclusion?	
What is best?	**Where do I find the information?**
The inclusion or exclusion of studies in a systematic review should be clearly defined a priori. The eligibility criteria used should specify the patients, interventions or exposures and outcomes of interest. In many cases the type of study design will also be a key component of the eligibility criteria.	The **Methods** section should describe in detail the inclusion and exclusion criteria. Normally, this will include the study design.

This paper: Yes ☐   No ☐   Unclear ☐   Comment: ....

Find — Did the search find all the relevant evidence?	
What is best?	**Where do I find the information?**
The starting point for a comprehensive search for all relevant studies is the major bibliographic databases (eg, MEDLINE, Cochrane, EMBASE) but should also include a search of reference lists from relevant studies, use of Science Citation Index, and contact with experts, particularly to inquire about unpublished studies. The search should not be limited to English language only. The search strategy should include both MeSH terms and text words.	The **Methods** section should describe the search strategy, including the terms used, in some detail. The **Results** section will outline the number of titles and abstracts reviewed, the number of full-text studies retrieved, and the number of studies excluded together with the reasons for exclusion. This information may be presented in a figure or flow chart.

This paper: Yes ☐   No ☐   Unclear ☐   Comment: ....

Appraise — Have the studies been critically appraised?

What is best?	Where do I find the information?
The article should describe how the quality of each study was assessed using predetermined quality criteria appropriate to the type of clinical question (eg, randomisation, blinding and completeness of follow-up for intervention questions).	The **Methods** section should describe the assessment of quality and the criteria used. The **Results** section should provide information on the quality of the individual studies.

This paper: Yes ☐   No ☐   Unclear ☐   Comment: ....

... and was the overall quality adequate?

What is best?	Where do I find the information?
The studies should be assessed independently by at least 2 reviewers. The overall quality should be such that the results are unlikely to be attributable to biases such as poor randomisation or unblinded subjects.	**Methods** section should describe how the assessments were done and by whom. The **Results** section should provide a table with information about the quality of the study and the likely degree of bias.

This paper: Yes ☐   No ☐   Unclear ☐   Comment: ....

Synthesise — Have the results been synthesised with appropriate summary tables and plots?

What is best?	Where do I find the information?
The results of included studies should at least be presented in a summary table. If the results are similar, there may be a meta-analysis with the results presented as a 'forest plot'. Ideally, this should also include a heterogeneity analysis (see below).	The **Results** section should include all the summary tables and plots and an explanation of the results.

This paper: Yes ☐   No ☐   Unclear ☐   Comment: ....

... and were the results similar between studies?

What is best?	Where do I find the information?
Ideally, the results of the different studies should be similar or homogeneous. If heterogeneity exists the authors may estimate whether the differences are significant (Cochrane Q test). Possible reasons for the heterogeneity should be explored.	The **Results** section should state whether the results are heterogeneous and discuss possible reasons. The forest plot should show the results of the Cochrane Q test for heterogeneity and discuss reasons for heterogeneity, if present.

This paper: Yes ☐   No ☐   Unclear ☐   Comment: ....

Step 3: What do the results mean?

What measure was used, how large was the effect (could it have been due to chance)?

Other comments

Papers

Parenteral metoclopramide for acute migraine: meta-analysis of randomised controlled trials

Ian Colman, Michael D Brown, Grant D Innes, Eric Grafstein, Ted E Roberts, Brian H Rowe

Abstract

Objective To assess the evidence from controlled trials on the efficacy and tolerability of parenteral metoclopramide for acute migraine in adults.

Data sources Cochrane Central Register of Controlled Trials, Medline, Embase, LILACS, CINAHL, conference proceedings, clinical practice guidelines, and other sources.

Selection criteria Randomised controlled trials of parenteral metoclopramide for acute migraine in adults.

Results We reviewed 596 potentially relevant abstracts and found 13 eligible trials totalling 655 adults. In studies comparing metoclopramide with placebo, metoclopramide was more likely to provide significant reduction in migraine pain (odds ratio 2.84, 95% confidence interval 1.05 to 7.68). Used as the only agent, metoclopramide showed mixed effectiveness when compared with other single agents. Heterogeneity of studies for combination treatment prevented statistical pooling. Treatments that did include metoclopramide were as, or more, effective than comparison treatments for pain, nausea, and relapse outcomes reported in all studies.

Conclusions Metoclopramide is an effective treatment for migraine headache and may be effective when combined with other treatments. Given its non-narcotic and antiemetic properties, metoclopramide should be considered a primary agent in the treatment of acute migraines in emergency departments.

Introduction

The pathophysiology of migraine is poorly understood, with no clear consensus on the best treatment for acute attacks. Current guidelines recommend agents such as sumatriptan, dihydroergotamine, ergotamine, chlorpromazine, and prochlorperazine.[1 2] Metoclopramide has long been used for the treatment of nausea associated with acute migraine. It also relieves gastric stasis and has the potential to enhance the absorption of other analgesics.[3] The dopamine antagonist properties of metoclopramide might make it effective as a single agent to treat acute migraine.[4] Other dopamine antagonists such as prochlorperazine and chlorpromazine have also shown effectiveness in migraine.[2]

We assessed the evidence from controlled trials on the efficacy and tolerability of parenteral metoclopramide for acute migraine in adults.

Methods

Our a priori study protocol is described elsewhere.[5] We searched the Cochrane Central Register of Controlled Trials, Medline, Embase, LILACS, and CINAHL using the search terms "headache" or "migraine" and "metoclopramide", "Maxeran", "Reglan", or "Maxolon".

To locate unpublished research, we reviewed proceedings from meetings on neurology, headache, and emergency medicine from 1998 to 2004, we assessed clinical practice guidelines, and we searched websites containing details of clinical trials, theses, or dissertations. We hand searched reference lists of all potentially relevant studies, and we contacted pharmaceutical companies, authors of previous studies, and experts in headache.

Studies were eligible for review if they were randomised controlled trials of parenteral metoclopramide given for acute migraine in adults, and described reasonable criteria to distinguish migraine from other headaches. We included trials conducted in a setting that indicated the headache was an acute episode—emergency department or headache clinic.

Study selection, data abstraction, and assessment of quality

Two independent reviewers (IC, EG) screened identified studies for eligibility. They reviewed the full manuscripts of potentially relevant papers for inclusion. Two independent reviewers (IC, MDB) abstracted information on to specially designed, pretested forms. Disagreements were resolved by consensus.

The internal validity of trials was assessed with the Jadad scale.[6] This evaluates quality of randomisation, blinding, and withdrawals and assigns a score from 0 to 5, higher scores indicating higher quality in the conduct or reporting of trials.

Department of Psychiatry, University of Cambridge, Cambridge
Ian Colman
postgraduate

Program in Emergency Medicine, Michigan State University, MI, 49503, USA
Michael D Brown
emergency physician

Department of Emergency Medicine, Providence Health Care and St Paul's Hospital, Vancouver, BC, Canada
Grant D Innes
emergency physician
Eric Grafstein
emergency physician

Department of Medicine, University of Alberta, Edmonton, AB, Canada
Ted E Roberts
neurologist

Division of Emergency Medicine, University of Alberta, 1G1.43 Walter Mackenzie Health Sciences Center, 8440-112 Street, Edmonton, AB, Canada T6G 2B7
Brian H Rowe
research director

Correspondence to:
B H Rowe
brian.rowe@
ualberta.ca

BMJ 2004;329:1369–72

Additional forest plots and details of excluded trials are on bmj.com

This is the abridged version of an article that was posted on bmj.com on 18 November 2004: http://bmj.com/cgi/doi/10.1136/bmj.38281.595718.7C

Reproduced with permission from BMJ Publishing Group Ltd.

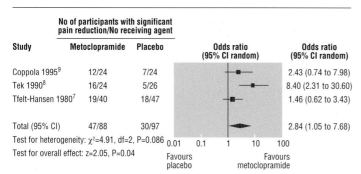

Study	No of participants with significant pain reduction/No receiving agent		Odds ratio (95% CI random)	Odds ratio (95% CI random)
	Metoclopramide	Placebo		
Coppola 1995[9]	12/24	7/24		2.43 (0.74 to 7.98)
Tek 1990[8]	16/24	5/26		8.40 (2.31 to 30.60)
Tfelt-Hansen 1980[7]	19/40	18/47		1.46 (0.62 to 3.43)
Total (95% CI)	47/88	30/97		2.84 (1.05 to 7.68)

Test for heterogeneity: χ^2=4.91, df=2, P=0.086
Test for overall effect: z=2.05, P=0.04

Fig 1 Metoclopramide compared with placebo for significant reduction in headache pain from acute migraine

We considered three outcomes describing relief of headache at the time closest to two hours after treatment. These were self reported as complete relief of headache, significant reduction in headache pain (from moderate or severe to mild or none), and reduction in headache pain using a visual analogue scale. Secondary outcomes included improvement in functional status or ability, relapse of migraine within 48 hours of treatment, reduction in nausea, number of co-intervention ("rescue") drugs required, and adverse events associated with treatment.

Statistical analysis and sensitivity analyses

Using random effects models, we pooled the results of studies, if appropriate, after consideration of heterogeneity between the trials. We tested for heterogeneity using a χ^2 test, with P values of less than 0.10 representing significance. Trials were not pooled when heterogeneity was evident and could be explained by dissimilarities in clinical variables. See bmj.com for details.

We completed our a priori sensitivity analyses comparing studies of high quality to those of low quality, based on the Jadad scale. These sensitivity analyses were only performed for outcomes reported in at least three studies.

Results

We identified 596 abstracts, of which 36 were potentially relevant articles. Independent review led to the inclusion of 13 studies (see bmj.com). As three of these studies had multiple arms, we were able to make 17 total comparisons. Study methods varied significantly, particularly for comparators and outcomes, and study quality was generally poor.

Metoclopramide versus placebo

Five studies (263 patients) compared metoclopramide with placebo. Metoclopramide was superior to placebo for all outcomes related to pain and nausea, although differences were not always statistically significant. Pooled data from three studies showed that metoclopramide more often led to significant reductions in headache pain (odds ratio 2.84, 95% confidence interval 1.05 to 7.68; fig 1), and in these studies, patients who received metoclopramide were significantly less likely to require rescue drugs (0.21, 0.05 to 0.85).[7-9] Three studies suggested that metoclopramide produced larger improvements in pain scores on a visual analogue scale, but no standard deviations were

reported, preventing statistical pooling. One study reported that metoclopramide was more likely than placebo to provide complete resolution of migraine; the difference, however, was not statistically significant (2.16, 0.36 to 12.84). Four studies found that metoclopramide was more effective than placebo in reducing nausea (4.20, 1.70 to 10.36), but only two studies reported relapse of migraine, and these found a statistically insignificant advantage favouring metoclopramide (0.30, 0.03 to 3.16).

Only two studies reported adverse events. One found a statistically insignificant increase in restlessness in the metoclopramide group (2.27, 0.19 to 26.81) whereas the other reported no restlessness, dystonic reactions, hypotension, or seizures in either treatment group.

Sensitivity analyses failed to identify differences between studies of high and low quality.

Metoclopramide versus other antiemetics

Three studies (194 patients) compared metoclopramide with other antiemetics (chlorpromazine and prochlorperazine). These suggested that metoclopramide was less effective in relieving pain and nausea, although differences were not always statistically significant. Two studies found no difference in the rate of complete resolution of migraine (0.64, 0.23 to 1.76) whereas two found that metoclopramide was less likely to provide significant relief of headache (0.39, 0.18 to 0.87); however, in one study, reduction in pain scores on a visual analogue scale was not different between groups (weighted mean difference -0.53, 95% confidence interval -1.63 to 0.57). Pooled results from all three studies showed that patients who received metoclopramide were more likely to require rescue drugs (odds ratio 2.08, 1.04 to 4.17). Two studies found no significant differences in relapse of migraine (3.95, 0.88 to 17.66). Metoclopramide was less effective than other antiemetics in reducing nausea, but these differences were not statistically significant.

Two studies looked at adverse events. One reported no restlessness, dystonic reactions, hypotension, or seizures in either treatment group, whereas the other described several subgroups of adverse events but found no statistically significant differences between groups.

Metoclopramide versus non-antiemetics

Two studies (60 patients) compared metoclopramide with non-antiemetics. The first found no significant differences between metoclopramide and sumatriptan in the rate of complete resolution of migraine (2.27, 0.64 to 8.11), the likelihood of significant reduction of pain (18.38 to 0.96, 352.59), or the likelihood of significant reduction of nausea (19.74, 1.00 to 390.32). In the second study, metoclopramide was compared with ibuprofen on the basis of scores to measure pain and nausea on a visual analogue scale. Metoclopramide produced larger decreases in scores for both outcomes, but standard deviations were not reported. Patients in the metoclopramide group were significantly less likely to require rescue drugs (0.05, 0.00 to 0.56). Neither study reported adverse events, no common outcomes were reported, and no statistical pooling was possible.

Reproduced with permission from BMJ Publishing Group Ltd.

Metoclopramide combinations versus other agents

Seven studies (211 patients) compared metoclopramide combinations (usually metoclopramide with dihydroergotamine) with other antimigraine regimens (hydroxyzine-meperidine, dihydroergotamine alone, valproate, ibuprofen, ketorolac, promethazine-meperidine). Owing to significant heterogeneity in study methods, studies were not pooled statistically.

One study showed that complete resolution of migraine was significantly more likely in patients who received metoclopramide (7.79, 1.79 to 33.86), and results from four studies suggested that patients who received metoclopramide were equally, or more, likely to have "significant reductions" in headache (fig 2).[10–13] Two studies showed that patients who received metoclopramide had equivalent, or larger, reductions in pain scores on the basis of a visual analogue scale (see fig A on bmj.com). We found no significant differences between groups for functional ability in two studies (see fig B on bmj.com) or nausea in two studies (see fig C on bmj.com). One study found no significant differences between groups in requirement for rescue drugs (0.22, 0.04 to 1.12). Three studies reported that patients who received metoclopramide were equally, or less, likely to have relapse of migraine (see fig D on bmj.com).

Reporting for adverse events was inconsistent. Four studies found no significant differences for nausea between groups. One study found restlessness, dysphoria, and flushing more common among patients treated with metoclopramide and dihydroergotamine than those treated with hydroxyzine and meperidine or butorphanol, and no significant differences for dizziness. Another study found that drowsiness, dizziness, and an orthostatic blood pressure response were less common among patients treated with metoclopramide and dihydroergotamine than those treated with promethazine and meperidine.

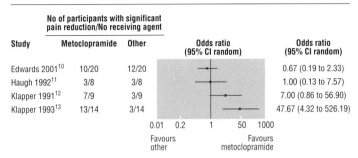

Fig 2 Metoclopramide combined with other agents compared with other agents for significant reduction in headache pain from acute migraine in adults

Discussion

Metoclopramide is an effective treatment for migraine headache in adults. Our systematic review suggests that as few as four patients need to be treated with metoclopramide to enable one patient to achieve a significant reduction in pain. Given its non-narcotic and antiemetic properties, metoclopramide should be considered as a primary agent in the treatment of acute migraine in emergency departments. Metoclopramide may, however, have less beneficial effects on nausea than other antiemetics.

Several studies scored less than 3 on the Jadad scale, undermining confidence in any conclusions drawn. It was difficult to combine the studies because of the many different comparators used and the many different outcomes reported.

Future trials should include multiple arms to compare various treatments under similar conditions, and there should be improvement in the quality of research. The International Headache Society's guidelines for controlled trials of drugs in migraine are a step in the right direction.[14]

Some of the trials did not report on inclusion and exclusion criteria in sufficient detail; consequently, we may have included studies of non-migraine headaches. Some failed to describe their study population, and most did not report initial severity and duration of headache. It is therefore possible we pooled studies with differing patient characteristics, so it is difficult to determine whether our results are generalisable.

Poor reporting of adverse events in most of the studies limits any conclusions about the relative safety of different agents, and the relatively small sample sizes provided insufficient power to detect meaningful differences in rates of uncommon adverse events.

Our study may have been affected by publication bias. However, we employed comprehensive search strategies to identify all relevant research. To avoid any selection bias, we used two independent reviewers and developed standardised criteria to identify and select studies for review.

We thank the Cochrane Library Pain, Palliative and Supportive Care Review Group for their guidance; Aventis Pharma for responding to our request for unpublished data; and study authors GL Ellis, J Jones, DS Tek, MJ Belgrade, KR Edwards, and JF Wilson. Data from this study were reported at the annual scientific meeting of the Canadian Association of Emergency Physicians, Winnipeg, Canada, June 2003 and will be maintained as a Cochrane Review in the Cochrane Library.

Contributors: See bmj.com

What is already known on this topic

Migraine headache is a common and disabling phenomenon that is not well understood

Parenteral metoclopramide is often given to relieve nausea associated with migraine headache

Metoclopramide may reduce pain associated with migraine headache

What this study adds

Parenteral metoclopramide is effective in reducing headache pain from acute migraine

As few as four patients need to be treated with metoclopramide to enable one additional patient to achieve significant reduction in pain

Parenteral metoclopramide may also be effective when combined with other treatments to enhance antimigraine effects

---

Reproduced with permission from BMJ Publishing Group Ltd.

Funding: This study was funded in part by the Division of Emergency Medicine, University of Alberta, Edmonton; the Canadian Institute of Health Research chairs programme, Ottawa; and the Canadian Association of Emergency Physicians Research Consortium, Ottawa.

Competing interests: BHR has received fees on two occasions from Aventis for speaking on venous thromboembolism. He has not been sponsored to speak on Maxeran or migraine headaches.

Ethical approval: Not required.

1   Silberstein SD. Practice parameter: evidence-based guidelines for migraine headache (an evidence-based review): report of the Quality Standards Subcommittee of the American Academy of Neurology. *Neurology* 2000;55:754-62.
2   Pryse-Phillips WE, Dodick DW, Edmeads JG, Gawel MJ, Nelson RF, Purdy RA, et al. Guidelines for the diagnosis and management of migraine in clinical practice. Canadian Headache Society. *CMAJ* 1997;156:1273-87.
3   Desmond PV, Watson KJR. Metoclopramide—a review. *Med J Aust* 1986;144:366-9.
4   Schwarzberg MN. Application of metoclopramide specificity in migraine attacks therapy. *Headache* 1994;34:439-41.
5   Colman I, Innes G, Brown MD, Roberts T, Grafstein E, Rowe BH. Parenteral metoclopramide for acute migraine. *Cochrane Database Syst Rev* 2003:CD003972.
6   Jadad AR, Moore RA, Carroll D, Jenkinson C, Reynolds DJ, Gavaghan DJ, et al. Assessing the quality of reports of randomized clinical trials: is blinding necessary? *Controlled Clin Trials* 1996;17:1-12.
7   Tfelt-Hansen P, Olesen J, Aebelholt-Krabbe A, Melgaard B, Veilis B. A double blind study of metoclopramide in the treatment of migraine attacks. *J Neurol Neurosurg Psychiatry* 1980;43:369-71.
8   Tek DS, McClellan DS, Olshaker JS, Allen CL, Arthur DC. A prospective, double-blind study of metoclopramide hydrochloride for the control of migraine in the emergency department. *Ann Emerg Med* 1990;19:1083-7.
9   Coppola M, Yealy DM, Leibold RA. Randomized, placebo-controlled evaluation of prochlorperazine versus metoclopramide for emergency department treatment of migraine headache. *Ann Emerg Med* 1995;26:541-6.
10 Edwards KR, Norton J, Behnke M. Comparison of intravenous valproate versus intramuscular dihydroergotamine and metoclopramide for acute treatment of migraine headache. *Headache* 2001;41:976-80.
11 Haugh MJ, Lavender L, Jensen LA, Giulano R. An office-based double-blind comparison of dihydroergotamine versus dihydroergotamine/metoclopramide in the treatment of acute migraine. *Headache* 1992;32:251.
12 Klapper JA, Stanton JS. Ketorolac versus DHE and metoclopramide in the treatment of migraine headaches. *Headache* 1991;31:523-4.
13 Klapper JA, Stanton JS. Current emergency treatment of severe migraine headaches. *Headache* 1993;33:560-2.
14 Tfelt-Hansen P, Block G, Dahlof C, Diener HC, Ferrari MD, Goadsby PJ, et al. Guidelines for controlled trials of drugs in migraine: second edition. *Cephalalgia* 2000;20:765-86.

(Accepted 6 October 2004)

doi 10.1136/bmj.38281.595718.7C

Reproduced with permission from BMJ Publishing Group Ltd.

Quiz: Critically appraise the evidence

1. When evaluating the internal validity of a randomised controlled trial the three most important things you would look for are (number the three most important as 1, 2, 3):

(a) Were all patients who entered the trial accounted for
     at its conclusion?   _____

(b) Are the inclusion criteria clearly stated?   _____

(c) Were the patients randomly selected from the
     target population?   _____

(d) Were the patients and clinicians kept blind as to which
     treatment was being received?   _____

(e) Was there a concealed randomisation list for
     allocating patients?   _____

(f) Were only patients who fully complied included in
     the final analysis?   _____

(g) Are the outcome measures clearly defined?   _____

2. When evaluating the internal validity of a systematic review the three most important things you would look for are (number the three most important as 1, 2, 3):

(a) Was there a well-defined question for the review?   _____

(b) Was the study question clearly linked to inclusion and
     exclusion criteria for the review?   _____

(c) Did the literature search cover enough sources to ensure
     that all relevant studies were retrieved?   _____

(d) Were the included studies critically appraised using
     appropriate quality criteria?   _____

(e) Were the included studies of sufficiently high quality
     that bias is unlikely?   _____

(f) Were the studies appraised by two reviewers?   _____

(g) Does the review include clear summary tables and
     plots to show the results?   _____

(h) Is there a heterogeneity analysis?   _____

Answers to this quiz are in the 'Answers' section in Part 4 of this workbook.

Notes

EBP Step 4: Apply the evidence

When you are satisfied that you have found the best evidence for your clinical question, either from a Cochrane systematic review, from another high-quality review or by critical appraisal of individual studies, the next step is to work out how the results of the search apply to your individual patient using your own clinical expertise and the values and preferences of the patient.

The questions that you should ask before you decide to apply the results of the study to your patient are:

▶ Is the treatment or test feasible in my setting?

▶ What else do I need to apply this evidence?

▶ What alternatives are available?

▶ Is my patient so different to those in the study that the results cannot apply at all?

▶ Will the potential benefits of treatment outweigh the potential harms of treatment for my patient?

▶ What does my patient think about it?

This application of evidence to individuals is sometimes called the 'external validity', or 'generalisability' of the research results.

Although this step is usually given as Step 4, which implies that it is done after Step 3 (Critically appraise the evidence), it is entirely up to you in which order you approach these two steps. For example, you will not want to waste time doing a critical appraisal of a study if it obviously will not apply or is infeasible in your clinical setting. On the other hand, you equally will not want to waste time working out the applicability of a study, only to find that it is a poor study. There is no easy answer to this — you will probably need to work it out on a case-by-case basis.

Is the treatment or test feasible in my setting?

You need to assess whether the treatment, diagnostic test or other factor described in the study would be feasible in your setting. Amongst the factors that you should consider are:

▶ Is the treatment or test available and practical in your setting?

> ### Steps in EBP
>
> 1. Formulate an answerable question.
>
> 2. Track down the best evidence of outcomes available.
>
> 3. Critically appraise the evidence (find out how good it is and what it means).
>
> 4. Apply the evidence (integrate the results with clinical expertise and patient values).

- ▶ Can you provide the necessary monitoring and follow-up required?

- ▶ Will your patient be willing and able to comply with the treatment regimen?

A particular problem with non-drug therapies is being able to replicate the treatment, as many studies do not provide a sufficiently detailed 'recipe' for us to be able to deliver the same treatment used in the trial. So if you and your colleagues are enthused by a new intervention, you may need to consider some homework such as writing to the author, investigating local options, or even getting the skills required to replicate the treatment.

What else do I need to apply this evidence?

In addition to the 'homework' mentioned above, you may also need more information about other types of studies, or to find out more about costs, or how many people are affected by the study findings. Alternatively, you may need to do a course or purchase some equipment. We call these actions 'next actions.' Sometimes you'll need to do several of them.

It is a good idea to keep a logbook of the questions you are asking and answering in clinical practice (see also 'How am I doing?', in Part 4 of this workbook). At the end of your logbook we suggest you should have specific sections for:

- ▶ the clinical bottom line, and

- ▶ 'next actions'.

You could also discuss these with others in your practice setting; for example, at your journal club meetings. In the box opposite are some examples of the type of 'next action' that might be needed.

It is useful to have group support in this process. If you haven't done so already, we strongly suggest setting up a regular 'clinical questions group' where you discuss current clinical problems with colleagues and use research evidence to help answer some of these. See the article by Phillips and Glasziou ('What makes evidence-based journal clubs succeed?') in the 'Further reading' section in Part 4 of this workbook.

> **Examples of 'next actions'**
>
> **Obtain more information**
>
> At a recent journal club we studied the use of combined long-acting beta-agonist and inhaled corticosteroid. The combination allowed patients to 'self-titrate' and looked promising compared to conventional alternatives. However, we wanted to check on other trials, on rumours we had heard about harms from long-acting beta-agonists, and on costs. Homework was assigned to do searches, find the costs, and email a local respiratory physician for information for discussion at our next meeting.
>
> **Find out more details about an intervention**
>
> We had critically appraised a systematic review of self-help cognitive behavioural therapy for the treatment of depression. This looked positive but lacked details on how it was done and what the books used were like. So we had two 'next actions': (i) to write to the review author for details about the interventions; and (ii) to get copies of some of the books used so we could look them over.
>
> So at our next journal club, one person brought along several of the books for us to look through, while another reported back that none of the 'self-help' was really book-only, but all had an element of follow-up support as well.
>
> **Audit those affected by the study results**
>
> Having critically appraised a systematic review in the *Lancet* suggesting atenolol was ineffective as an antihypertensive (it lowered blood pressure but not cardiovascular events), we decided we should check how many patients were on atenolol and what they were on it for. In addition, we sought further information about alternatives before deciding what to do as a practice.

What alternatives are there?

If there are other alternative treatments or procedures that you could use, then you need to weigh up which one would be most suitable for your patient, balancing the potential benefits and harms of each option. Is doing nothing an option? (This relies on your interpretation of the benefits and risks of harm for your patient and on what the patient thinks; see below.)

Is my patient sufficiently similar to those in the study?

As your patients were not in the studies you have researched, you need to use your clinical expertise to decide whether they are sufficiently similar to the subjects in the studies for the results to be applicable to them. The crucial factor that may affect your decision is the nature of your patient's illness — the severity or stage or degree of risk — and whether it matches the subjects in the studies. Other patient features may also be important such as:

▶ age (the clinical trials may have older adults but your patients may be over 80)

▶ comorbidity (your patient may have another condition and be taking drugs that could interact with the one tested in the trial)

▶ likely compliance (you may feel that your patient is unlikely to comply with the regimen because of other factors).

These factors will tell you if your patient is at higher risk than the trial subjects (and likely to benefit more than those in the trial), or at lower risk than the trial subjects (and therefore likely to benefit less).

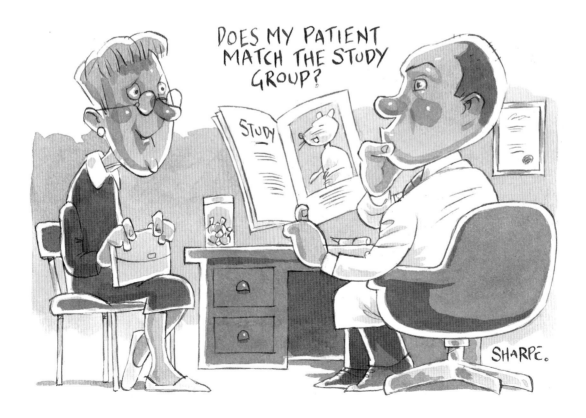

Will the potential benefits outweigh the potential harms of treatment for my patient?

If possible from the study results, work out the number needed to treat (NNT) and, for adverse effects, the number needed to harm (NNH).

You then need to estimate your patient's risk of the outcome in question, which may be higher or lower than the control group in the study. The general problem is illustrated in the figure below. In general the benefit of treatment will increase with the risk or severity of illness (except at extremes), but the harms will usually not change with the degree of risk or severity. So once a patient is sufficiently at risk or their condition is sufficiently severe, treatment is worth the possible harms from treatment. Therefore there is a risk threshold above which treatment has a net worth. As Hippocrates (almost) said: *'Firstly, do no net harm'.*

For a positive trial (see figure below), the trial patients (i) will show this net benefit. However, our patient may be at lower risk (ii) and hence treatment is now worthwhile, or at higher risk (iii) and hence treatment is even more worthwhile. In general primary care patients will have lower risk or less severe illness than secondary care patients. So fewer will benefit from treatment. But this is an individual problem, not a setting problem: some patients in primary care may still benefit more than the average secondary care patient.

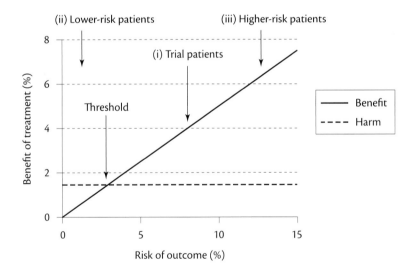

A shortcut you may like to use is to estimate the study NNT and NNH in line with your patients' personal risk factors using a method called the 'f method'.

> **The 'f method' for estimating your patient's risk:**
>
> If your patient is twice as susceptible as those in the trial, f = 2
>
> If your patient is half as susceptible as those in the trial, f = 0.5
>
> Assuming the treatment produces the same relative risk reduction for patients at different levels of risk, then:
>
> the NNT for your patient = NNT (trial)/f
>
> References:
>
> Glasziou PP, Irwig LM (1995). An evidence based approach to individualising treatment. *British Medical Journal* 311(7016):1356–1359.
>
> Sackett DL, Straus SE, Richardson WS et al (2000). *Evidence-Based Medicine: How to Practice and Teach EBM*, Churchill Livingstone.

If the NNTs are similar for different treatments, look at the NNH for harmful side-effects and choose the treatment with least side-effects (this will also increase compliance).

What does my patient think about the options?

It is important to understand and consider what the patient thinks, once you have explained the risks and benefits of different treatment options. The outcomes that are important to you may not be those that are important to the patient, particularly where quality of life is concerned (for example, if compliance with the treatment is onerous or there are adverse effects).

A simple communication process to explain natural history and integrate it with decision about treatment can be guided by the following three steps:

1. What would happen if we did nothing?

You might begin by saying something like: 'Do you know about X? OK, well let me explain. If we did nothing the usual course of the illness is to ...'

2. Explain what the options are

Next list and explain the main management options, for example: 'There are three common things we can do about this: a pill, or surgery, or we can let it take its course (natural history)'.

3. Check the patient's expectations and ideas

We should know if the patient has tried any of the options, or has prior knowledge and expectations about them. For example, you could ask: 'Have you tried anything yourself, or do you have a preference for one of those options?' At this point a dialogue may ensue about the pros and cons of the various options, or the patient may simply ask what you recommend.

References:

Del Mar C, Doust J, Glasziou P (2006). *Clinical Thinking: Evidence, Communication and Decision Making*, BMJ Books, Blackwell Publishing Ltd, London.

NHMRC Working Committee on Communicating the Risks, Benefits and Outcomes of Elective Therapy (Dr Peter Greenberg, Chair) (2006). *Making Decisions about Tests and Treatments: Principles for Better Communication Between Healthcare Consumers and Healthcare Professionals*, National Health and Medical Research Council, Australian Government, Canberra. http://www.nhmrc.gov.au/publications/synopses/hpr25syn.htm

Quiz: Applying the evidence

1. In the trial of a new drug, Wundamycin, the mortality rate was 9% compared to 13% in the placebo group. How many similar patients need to be treated to prevent one death?

2. If you had a patient who was at lower risk (you estimate 3%) but the relative effects of Wundermycin were the same, what would be the expected absolute risk reduction and number needed to treat?

3. Joan has had an uneventful recovery from hospitalisation, but 2 weeks later is now seeing you, her GP, for a follow-up check. She asks about what role diet has in 'heart disease'. She asks specifically about a 'Mediterranean' diet, which one of the nurses in Coronary Care had mentioned to her.

(Continued on page 140)

Read and appraise the abstract below and use it to answer the following questions:

   a. What are the strengths and weaknesses of this study? Do you think these results are valid? Explain.

   b. The risk ratio is said to be 0.27 – explain what this means.

   c. Calculate the absolute risk reduction and the number needed to treat (NNT).

   d. What advice would you give Joan based on this article?

ABSTRACT [de Lorgeril M, et al (1994). Mediterranean alpha-linolenic acid-rich diet in secondary prevention of coronary heart disease. *Lancet* 343(8911): 1454–1459.]

In a prospective, randomised single-blinded secondary prevention trial we compared the effect of a Mediterranean alpha-linolenic acid-rich diet to the usual post-infarct prudent diet. After a first myocardial infarction, patients were randomly assigned to the experimental ($n = 302$) or control group ($n = 303$). Patients were seen again 8 weeks after randomisation, and each year for 5 years.

The experimental group consumed significantly less lipids, saturated fat, cholesterol, and linoleic acid but more oleic and alpha-linolenic acids confirmed by measurements in plasma. Serum lipids, blood pressure, and body mass index remained similar in the 2 groups. In the experimental group, plasma levels of albumin, vitamin E, and vitamin C were increased, and granulocyte count decreased. After a mean follow up of 27 months, there were 16 cardiac deaths in the control and 3 in the experimental group; 17 non-fatal myocardial infarction in the control and 5 in the experimental groups: a risk ratio for these two main endpoints combined of 0.27 (95% CI 0.12 to 0.59, $P = 0.001$) after adjustment for prognostic variables. Overall mortality was 20 in the control, 8 in the experimental group, an adjusted risk ratio of 0.30 (95% CI 0.11 to 0.82, $P = 0.02$).

An alpha-linolenic acid-rich Mediterranean diet seems to be more efficient than presently used diets in the secondary prevention of coronary events and death.

Answers to this quiz are in the 'Answers' section in Part 4 of this workbook.

Part 3

Further critical appraisal exercises

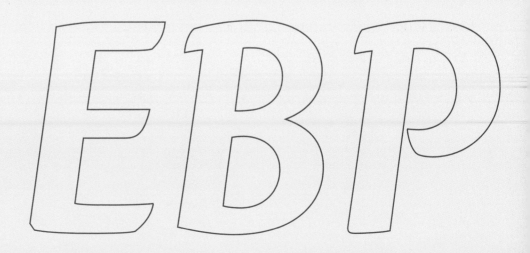

Critical appraisal of studies for a prognosis question

In EBP Step 1 (Formulate an answerable question) we saw how the PICO method of formulating a health care question can be used for questions about aetiology and risk factors, frequency and rate, and prognosis (population/ problem, intervention/indicator, control, outcome). As we saw in the table of levels of evidence on page 42, it is not necessary to do randomised controlled trials (RCTs) to answer frequency and rate, or prognosis questions. Furthermore, although it is possible to do randomised studies to answer aetiology questions, it is often impractical or not ethical. Therefore, for these question types, the study designs that you are likely to find are observational studies, such as case–control studies, cohort studies or cross-sectional studies (see EBP Step 2: Track down the best evidence, and the Glossary, for further information about these types of studies).

So, if your question was about aetiology and risk factors, frequency or rate, or prognosis you may have found a cohort study or a case–control study. How can you tell if the results are reliable? Once again, we turn to critical appraisal using the same principles that we have already discussed for RCTs:

▶   Question 1: How well does the PICO of the study match your PICO?

▶   Question 2: How well was the study done (RAMMbo)?

▶   Question 3: What do the results mean?

In this section, we will focus on studies that answer a prognosis question. We will not walk you through a paper in detail but ask you to go straight ahead and try appraising one yourself using the boxes below. Some suggested 'answers' are in the 'Answers' section in Part 4 of this workbook. To set the scene, imagine that you see a retired female patient who has previously had a venous thromboembolism (VT) that was treated with anticoagulants. She wants to know her chances of having another VT. You know that the incidence of a first VT is different for men and women at different ages but you do not know what the recurrence rate is for men and women.

In other words, your clinical question is:

P   *For adults who have had a previous VT...*

I/C   *... is there a difference between men (I) and women (C)*

O   *... in the risk of a further VT?*

Your search on PubMed has identified an article about the risk of recurrent VT in men and women:

> Kyrle et al (2004). The risk of recurrent venous thromboembolism in men and women. *New England Journal of Medicine* 350:2558–2563.
> (The full article is included on pages 152–157 of this workbook.)

The methods section of the paper shows that it is a cohort study, so you wonder how reliable the results are.

Question 1: How well does the PICO of the study match your PICO?

As we have already seen in EBP Step 3 (Critically appraise the evidence), it is a good idea to work out the PICO of your paper to see whether it matches your PICO. In the case of prognosis studies, there are two types of question. First, there may be a simple 'PO' question, which asks about the outcome of a particular condition:

P   *For adults with a history of <a condition>...*

O   *... what is the risk of <an outcome>?*

This is a crucial initial question. But we may also wish to know whether the prognosis varies with different factors or indicators, such as whether gender affects the prognosis, as in the case of your clinical question about VT.

What is the PICO of the VT study?

Question 2: How well was the study done?

The steps for assessing how well a prognostic research study (cohort study) has been done (internal validity) follow the RAMMbo principle for primary research studies. However, in the case of a prognostic study, there is no random allocation to treatment; instead we must be wary of how treatment may have altered the natural history (for our PO question) or the relationship between a prognostic indicator and the outcome (our PICO question). The main features to look out for are described below.

RAMMbo to the rescue

Recruitment

As for all primary studies, the subjects in prognostic studies should be representative of the population that is the subject of the research question. Essentially, as for any research, the results of observational studies can only be extrapolated to a population with similar characteristics to those of the population studied. Therefore, if the population studied includes only a subset of the wider population (such as men, smokers, or a specific ethnic group), the results will only directly apply to that subset.

The research questions addressed by observational studies tend to be broader (more population-based) questions than for RCTs, with multiple variables and confounding factors. Great care is therefore needed to create well-defined and representative samples.

Good-quality prognostic (and other observational) studies have a well-defined research question and include a large number of people with carefully defined characteristics relating to the research question. Ideally, a consecutive or random sample of subjects should be selected at a similar time point with respect to the condition of interest. If this time point is at the beginning of the disease or other health condition, this is called an '**inception cohort**'.

> **Recruitment — How were the subjects in the VT study recruited?**

145

Adjustment

For observational studies, allocation to groups (such as exposures or prognostic indicators) is not random. For a cohort study, a study group (cohort) of people who have received a specific treatment, have been exposed to a particular situation (such as a risk factor for disease), or have a particular characteristic (indicator), is followed forward in time and compared with a matched group who either are not exposed (controls) or have a defined different exposure or characteristic of interest. For a case–control study, the previous exposure of people with a specific outcome is traced back and compared with the background of people without the outcome.

For the simple PO question about natural history, adjustment may be needed if some patients are treated (either initially or during the follow-up period). For PICO questions about the effect of a prognostic indicator, we need to take particular care about adjustment for treatment so that we don't suggest something as a risk factor when it is just a marker for treatment. We may also be interested in the independent contribution of a new risk factor over other known prognostic factors, in which case we will need to adjust for those other factors. This adjustment may be done by stratification or multivariate statistical methods, such as logistic or Cox regression analysis.

> ### Adjustment — How were the results of the VT study adjusted to make the groups comparable?
>
> ....
>
> ....
>
> ....
>
> ....

Maintenance

There are two important elements here. First, the study subjects should be maintained on the same non-treatment (for natural history) or treatment (for treatment-related prognosis) for the duration of the study. If this is not possible, appropriate statistical adjustments may be needed (see 'Adjustment' above). For treatment cohorts, the initial and subsequent treatment should be clearly spelt out, and an assessment given of the likely impact of this treatment on the 'natural history' of illness without treatment.

Second, a sufficient proportion of patients should be followed for long enough to detect the outcome of interest (eg for pregnancy outcomes, nine months; for cancer, many years). We usually ask for more than 80% of subjects to be followed up. Reasons for loss to follow-up should be provided along with the characteristics of those patients.

Maintenance — How were the study groups in the VT study managed and followed up?

....

....

....

....

Measurement

As allocation to groups is not random for observational studies, it is not possible to conceal allocation from the subjects. However, whenever possible, the outcomes should be measured by independent assessors who do not know (ie are blind) to the prognostic factors of the subjects (such as high cholesterol, smoking, or exposure to an environmental chemical). As for RCTs, this blinding is less important if an objective outcome is used (ie one that is not subject to the bias of the assessor).

> **Measurement — How were the outcomes of the VT study measured?**
>
> ....
>
> ....
>
> ....
>
> ....

Question 3: What do the results mean?

The results of prognostic studies are similar to the results of RCTs and many of the same considerations apply. That is, the difference between the groups studied may be expressed either as a continuous (such as height or weight) or non-continuous (develops disease or not) outcome with confidence intervals. Non-continous outcomes are also expressed as risk reductions.

A useful way of presenting risk information is as a 'survival curve', which shows how events occurred over the time course of the study. The figure opposite shows the recurrence of VT in the paper we are appraising. It plots the cumulative percentage of subjects with a VT event against time.

Likelihood of recurrent venous thromboembolism by sex

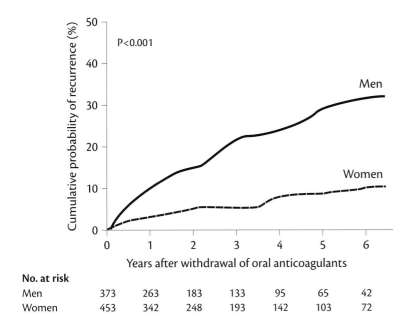

No. at risk

Men	373	263	183	133	95	65	42
Women	453	342	248	193	142	103	72

From the survival curves in the figure above, we can see that men have around a 9% recurrence of VT within 1 year, 18% within 2 years, and about 30% by 5 years. We can also see that the cumulative percentage of women with a recurrence was much lower than for men (and that this difference was statistically significant with $P < 0.001$). For both men and women, the risk seems slightly higher early on, after which there is a steady linear rise over time. If we just take the 5-year time point, there are several ways we can compare the sexes. The men have an absolute risk (AR) of around 30% whereas the women have an AR of around 8%. So the absolute risk difference is 30 − 8 = 22%; whereas the relative risk is 30/8 = 3.75 (375%). As we have already seen in Part 2, Step 3 of this workbook, the relative risk is a ratio of risks (for which there are two closely related measures: the odds ratio and the hazard ratio).

Part of the increased risk in men is attributable to the fact that they were older (51 versus 45 years), and so the paper has adjusted the relative risk for this, but it is still 3.4 after adjustment. In general, when there are several risk factors (prognostic indicators), it is helpful to see the individual contribution of each. The VT study shows the influence of the prognostic indicator both in isolation ('univariate') and in conjunction with all the other factors ('multivariate'). This is shown in the table on page 150. Factor IX looks like a moderately influential factor in isolation (relative risk [RR] of 1.8 with a confidence interval [CI] that does not cross 1), but less so when considered together with all the other factors (RR of 1.3 and a CI that crosses 1).

Relative risk of recurrent venous thromboembolism according to baseline characteristics

Characteristic	Univariate relative risk (95% CI)	Multivariate relative risk (95% CI)[a]
Age (per 10-year increase)	1.2 (1.1–1.4)	1.1 (0.9–1.3)
Symptomatic pulmonary embolism (vs deep vein thrombosis)	1.7 (1.2–2.5)	1.7 (1.1–2.5)
Factor V Leiden (vs absence of mutation)	1.0 (0.7–1.6)	1.2 (0.8–1.8)
Factor II G20210A (vs absence of mutation)	1.7 (0.9–3.1)	2.1 (1.1–3.8)
Factor VIII >234 IU/dL (vs <234 IU/dL)	3.4 (2.1–5.6)	2.9 (1.6–5.1)
Factor IX >138 IU/dL (vs <138 IU/dL)	1.8 (1.2–2.7)	1.3 (0.8–2.0)
Duration of anticoagulation (per 3-month increase)	1.03 (0.99–1.07)	1.02 (0.98–1.05)

CI, confidence interval.

[a] Multivariate relative risks were calculated with adjustment for age; the presence or absence of a first symptomatic pulmonary embolism, factor V Leiden, factor II G20210A, elevated factor VIII levels, or elevated factor IX levels; and the duration of anticoagulation.

One final point to note is the number of patients followed, as shown in the figure on the previous page as the 'No. at risk'. There are three ways the numbers can decrease:

▶ if a subject has an event

▶ if a subject is lost to follow-up

▶ if a subject has reached their maximum duration of follow-up.

The latter will be different for different subjects: those recruited early will have longer follow-up than those recruited nearer the end.

Now try to answer the following questions (answers are in the back of the book).

What do the results of the VT study mean?

1. In men, what is the risk of recurrence at (a) 1 year and (b) 5 years?

   ....

2. What is the difference in risk between men and women at 3 years (expressed in terms of absolute and relative risk)?

   ....

3. How many years before 20% of men have had a recurrence?

   ....

Summary of the critical appraisal of the VT study

R ....

A ....

M ....

M **b** **o** ....

Results ....

....

Overall ....

....

The NEW ENGLAND JOURNAL of MEDICINE

ORIGINAL ARTICLE

The Risk of Recurrent Venous Thromboembolism in Men and Women

Paul A. Kyrle, M.D., Erich Minar, M.D., Christine Bialonczyk, M.D., Mirko Hirschl, M.D., Ansgar Weltermann, M.D., and Sabine Eichinger, M.D.

ABSTRACT

From the Department of Internal Medicine I, Division of Hematology and Hemostasis (P.A.K., A.W., S.E.), Ludwig Boltzmann-Institut für Thromboseforschung (P.A.K.), and the Department of Internal Medicine II, Division of Angiology, Medical University of Vienna (E.M.); Wilhelminenspital (C.B.); and Hanusch Krankenhaus (M.H.) — all in Vienna. Address reprint requests to Dr. Kyrle at the Department of Internal Medicine I, Division of Hematology and Hemostasis, Währinger Gürtel 18-20, A 1090 Vienna, Austria, or at paul.kyrle@meduniwien.ac.at.

N Engl J Med 2004;350:2558-63.
Copyright © 2004 Massachusetts Medical Society.

BACKGROUND

Whether a patient's sex is associated with the risk of recurrent venous thromboembolism is unknown.

METHODS

We studied 826 patients for an average of 36 months after a first episode of spontaneous venous thromboembolism and the withdrawal of oral anticoagulants. We excluded pregnant patients and patients with a deficiency of antithrombin, protein C, or protein S; the lupus anticoagulant; cancer; or a requirement for potentially long-term antithrombotic treatment. The end point was objective evidence of a recurrence of symptomatic venous thromboembolism.

RESULTS

Venous thromboembolism recurred in 74 of the 373 men, as compared with 28 of the 453 women (20 percent vs. 6 percent; relative risk of recurrence, 3.6; 95 percent confidence interval, 2.3 to 5.5; P<0.001). The risk remained unchanged after adjustment for age, the duration of anticoagulation, and the presence or absence of a first symptomatic pulmonary embolism, factor V Leiden, factor II G20210A, or an elevated level of factor VIII or IX. At five years, the likelihood of recurrence was 30.7 percent among men, as compared with 8.5 percent among women (P<0.001). The relative risk of recurrence was similar among women who had had their first thrombosis during oral-contraceptive use or hormone-replacement therapy and women in the same age group in whom the first event was idiopathic.

CONCLUSIONS

The risk of recurrent venous thromboembolism is higher among men than women.

Downloaded from www.nejm.org at OXFORD UNIVERSITY LIBRARY SERVICES on May 8, 2006 .
Copyright © 2004 Massachusetts Medical Society. All rights reserved.

Reproduced with permission from Massachusetts Medical Society.

152

THE ANNUAL INCIDENCE OF VENOUS thromboembolism is 1 to 2 cases per 1000 persons,[1,2] and the risk of the disorder rises exponentially with age, from an annual rate of less than 5 per 100,000 children to greater than 400 per 100,000 adults older than 80 years.[3] The overall incidence of a first venous thromboembolism seems to be similar among men and women,[1-3] but the risk is higher among women of childbearing age than among men in the same age group.[2,4,5] This difference probably relates to the association of venous thromboembolism with pregnancy or the use of oral contraceptives. By contrast, the risk among older women is substantially lower than that among men in the same age group.[2,4,5]

Venous thromboembolism has a recurrence rate of 5 to 10 percent per year.[6-8] As for a first episode, the pathogenesis of recurrences is multifactorial, with risks that depend on the severity and number of hereditary and circumstantial factors. Whether a patient's sex is associated with the risk of recurrent venous thromboembolism is uncertain. Large prospective studies of the incidence of recurrence did not address sex.[6,8] In a study in Norway,[7] proximal deep-vein thrombosis, cancer, and a history of venous thromboembolism, but not the person's sex, predicted an increased risk of recurrent thrombotic events. In this report, we assessed the association of patient sex with the risk of recurrence in 826 patients with a first episode of spontaneous venous thromboembolism.

METHODS

PATIENTS AND STUDY DESIGN

The Austrian Study on Recurrent Venous Thromboembolism is an ongoing prospective study involving four thrombosis centers in Vienna. Between July 1992 and June 2003, 2795 patients older than 18 years of age who had been treated with oral anticoagulants for at least three months after venous thromboembolism were enrolled after providing written informed consent. All patients had been treated with standard heparin at doses designed to keep the activated partial-thromboplastin time 1.5 to 2.0 times that of the control value or with subcutaneous low-molecular-weight heparin at therapeutic doses. A total of 1945 patients were excluded because of the following conditions: previous venous thromboembolism in 451; surgery, trauma, or pregnancy within the previous three months in 527; a known deficiency of antithrombin, protein C, or protein S in 65; the lupus anticoagulant in 43; can-

cer in 423; and the need for long-term treatment with antithrombotic drugs for reasons other than venous thrombosis in 436.

The day of discontinuation of oral anticoagulants was defined as the day of study entry. After three weeks, patients were screened for the presence of a deficiency of antithrombin, protein C, and protein S; the lupus anticoagulant; factor V Leiden; and factor II G20210A. Levels of factors VIII and IX were also determined. The 24 patients who had a deficiency of antithrombin, protein C, or protein S or in whom the lupus anticoagulant was detected were excluded. Patients were observed at three-month intervals for the first year and every six months thereafter. They were provided with detailed written information on the symptoms of venous thromboembolism and were instructed to report to one of the thrombosis centers in case of symptoms. All women were strongly discouraged from using contraceptive pills or hormone-replacement therapy regardless of whether they had a history of an association between the use of these hormones and the initial venous thromboembolism. At each visit, a data form was completed regarding the patient's medical history.

DIAGNOSIS OF VENOUS THROMBOEMBOLISM

The diagnosis of deep-vein thrombosis was established by venography or color-coded duplex sonography (in the case of proximal deep-vein thrombosis). If venography was used, one of the following direct or indirect criteria had to be fulfilled: a constant filling defect was present on two views; there was an abrupt discontinuation of the contrast-filled vessel at a constant point in the vein; and the entire deep-vein system failed to fill without an external compressing process, with or without venous flow through collateral veins. Diagnostic criteria for color-coded duplex sonography were the following: visualization of an intraluminal thrombus in a deep vein, lack of or incomplete compressibility, and lack of flow spontaneously and after distal manipulation. The diagnosis of pulmonary embolism was made by ventilation–perfusion lung scanning according to the criteria of the Prospective Investigation of Pulmonary Embolism Diagnosis.[9] Patients with both deep-vein thrombosis and pulmonary embolism were categorized as having pulmonary embolism.

OUTCOME MEASURES

The end point of the study was recurrence of symptomatic venous thromboembolism confirmed by

Downloaded from www.nejm.org at OXFORD UNIVERSITY LIBRARY SERVICES on May 8, 2006 .
Copyright © 2004 Massachusetts Medical Society. All rights reserved.

Reproduced with permission from Massachusetts Medical Society.

venography, ventilation–perfusion lung scanning, or both, according to the aforementioned criteria. The diagnosis was established by an adjudication committee consisting of independent clinicians and radiologists who were aware of the patient's sex but unaware of the presence or absence of thrombotic risk factors. Recurrent deep-vein thrombosis was diagnosed if the patient had a thrombus in another deep vein in the leg involved in the previous event, a thrombus in the other leg, or a thrombus in the same venous system involved in the previous event with a proximal extension of the thrombus if the upper limit of the original thrombus had been visible or the presence of a constant filling defect surrounded by contrast medium if it had not.

LABORATORY ANALYSIS

Venous blood was obtained after the patient had fasted overnight, placed in 1/10 volume of 0.11 mmol of trisodium citrate per liter, and centrifuged for 20 minutes at 2000×g. The plasma was stored at –80°C. Routine laboratory methods were used to identify antithrombin, protein C, and protein S. Screening for factor V Leiden and factor II G20210A was carried out on genomic DNA as described previously.[10,11] Factor VIII and factor IX were measured by one-step clotting assays with the use of factor VIII– or factor IX–deficient plasma (Immuno Baxter) and a Sysmex CA 6000 fully automated coagulation analyzer. The presence of the lupus anticoagulant was established on the basis of the criteria of the Subcommittee on Lupus Anticoagulant/Antiphospholipid Antibody of the Scientific and Standardisation Committee of the International Society on Thrombosis and Haemostasis.[12] The technicians were unaware of the patient's characteristics, including sex, at all times.

STATISTICAL ANALYSIS

Categorical data were compared between groups with use of contingency-table analyses (the chi-square test), and continuous data (presented as means ±SD) were compared with use of Mann–Whitney U tests. All P values were two-tailed. Survival-time methods were used to analyze the time to recurrent venous thromboembolism among patients with a subsequent episode (uncensored observations) or the duration of follow-up among patients without recurrence (censored observations).[13] The probability of recurrence was estimated according to the method of Kaplan and Meier.[14] Data on patients who left the study because of a require-ment for potentially long-term antithrombotic treatment, a diagnosis of cancer, or pregnancy, who were lost to follow-up, or who died were censored at the time of withdrawal. To test for homogeneity among the various groups of patients, we used the log-rank test. Univariate and multivariate Cox proportional-hazards models were used to analyze the association of the patient's sex with the risk of recurrent venous thromboembolism. Analyses were adjusted for age, the presence or absence of symptomatic pulmonary embolism at the time of a first thrombotic event, the duration of anticoagulation, and the presence or absence of factor V Leiden, factor II G20210A, and elevated levels of factors VIII and IX (dichotomized at the 90th percentile [234 IU per deciliter] and at the 75th percentile [138 IU per deciliter] of the patient population, respectively). All computations were performed with the use of SPSS software, version 10.0.

RESULTS

STUDY POPULATION

We studied 826 patients (373 men and 453 women) who had had a first episode of spontaneous venous thromboembolism. The mean ages of these men and women were 51±14 years and 45±18 years, respectively (P<0.001). They were enrolled after the discontinuation of oral anticoagulants and followed for a median of 26 months. The median duration of follow-up was 23 months (interquartile range, 10 to 49) among the men and 28 months (interquartile range, 12 to 57) among the women (P=0.02). A total of 189 patients left the study: 125 required long-term antithrombotic treatment for reasons other than venous thromboembolism (15 women and 10 men received anticoagulants because of atrial fibrillation and 54 women and 46 men were given aspirin for arterial disease), 14 received a diagnosis of cancer, 26 became pregnant and started prophylaxis with low-molecular-weight heparin, and 24 were lost to follow-up. Three patients died of cancer, six of cardiac failure, and one of septicemia.

RECURRENT VENOUS THROMBOEMBOLISM

A total of 102 of the 826 patients (12 percent) had recurrent venous thromboembolism (deep-vein thrombosis in 67 and pulmonary embolism in 35). Of these 102 patients, 74 (73 percent) were men and 28 (27 percent) were women. Table 1 shows the relative risk of a recurrence according to age, the presence of a previous symptomatic pulmonary

Downloaded from www.nejm.org at OXFORD UNIVERSITY LIBRARY SERVICES on May 8, 2006 .
Copyright © 2004 Massachusetts Medical Society. All rights reserved.

Reproduced with permission from Massachusetts Medical Society.

embolism, factor V Leiden, factor II G20210A, or an elevated level of factor VIII or IX, and the duration of anticoagulation. When age was analyzed in a Cox proportional-hazards model, the relative risk of recurrent venous thromboembolism was 1.2 (95 percent confidence interval, 1.1. to 1.4; P=0.001) for each 10-year increase and 1.1 (95 percent confidence interval, 0.9 to 1.3; P=0.3) in the multivariate analysis. An elevated level of factor VIII and a first symptomatic pulmonary embolism were the strongest determinants of recurrence.

RECURRENT VENOUS THROMBOEMBOLISM AND SEX

Venous thromboembolism recurred in 74 of the 373 men, as compared with 28 of the 453 women (20 percent vs. 6 percent, P<0.001). Table 2 shows the baseline characteristics of all patients. The men were on average older than the women (51±14 years vs. 45±18 years, P<0.001), and they had a shorter duration of follow-up (33±29 months vs. 38±33 months, P=0.02). There was no significant difference between men and women with regard to the presence of factor V Leiden (31 percent and 29 percent, respectively), factor II G20210A (7 percent and 8 percent, respectively), elevated levels of factor VIII (8 percent and 10 percent, respectively), elevated levels of factor IX (25 percent and 22 percent, respectively), or the duration of anticoagulation (eight months and nine months, respectively). According to Kaplan–Meier analysis, there was a clear divergence between the rate of recurrence among men and the rate among women throughout the period of observation (P<0.001) (Fig. 1). At five years, the cumulative probability of recurrence was 30.7 percent (95 percent confidence interval, 23.8 to 37.6) among men, as compared with 8.5 percent (95 percent confidence interval, 5.0 to 12.0) among women. According to the univariate analysis, male sex conferred a relative risk of recurrence of 3.6 (95 percent confidence interval, 2.3 to 5.5; P<0.001). After adjustments for age, the duration of anticoagulation, and the presence or absence of a first symptomatic pulmonary embolism, factor V Leiden, factor II G20210A, and an elevated level of factor VIII or IX, the risk of recurrence among men, as compared with women, was 3.6 (95 percent confidence interval, 2.3 to 5.8; P<0.001).

A first venous thromboembolism occurred during oral-contraceptive use in 175 women. The cumulative probability of recurrence at five years was 5.9 percent (95 percent confidence interval, 0.6 to

11.1) among these women and 4.3 percent (95 percent confidence interval, 0 to 10.1; P=0.8) among the 60 women in the same age groups in whom the first event was idiopathic (Fig. 2). Among women who were taking oral contraceptives, the relative risk of recurrence was 0.8 (95 percent confidence interval, 0.1 to 4.0; P=0.8) and remained unchanged after adjustment for age and other possibly confounding factors.

Table 1. Relative Risk of Recurrent Venous Thromboembolism According to Baseline Characteristics.*

Characteristic	Univariate Relative Risk (95% CI)	Multivariate Relative Risk (95% CI)†
Age (per 10-yr increase)	1.2 (1.1–1.4)	1.1 (0.9–1.3)
Symptomatic pulmonary embolism (vs. deep-vein thrombosis)	1.7 (1.2–2.5)	1.7 (1.1–2.5)
Factor V Leiden (vs. absence of mutation)	1.0 (0.7–1.6)	1.2 (0.8–1.8)
Factor II G20210A (vs. absence of mutation)	1.7 (0.9–3.1)	2.1 (1.1–3.8)
Factor VIII ≥234 IU/dl (vs. <234 IU/dl)	3.4 (2.1–5.6)	2.9 (1.6–5.1)
Factor IX ≥138 IU/dl (vs. <138 IU/dl)	1.8 (1.2–2.7)	1.3 (0.8–2.0)
Duration of anticoagulation (per 3-mo increase)	1.03 (0.99–1.07)	1.02 (0.98–1.05)

* CI denotes confidence interval.
† Multivariate relative risks were calculated with adjustment for age; the presence or absence of a first symptomatic pulmonary embolism, factor V Leiden, factor II G20210A, elevated factor VIII levels, or elevated factor IX levels; and the duration of anticoagulation.

Table 2. Baseline Characteristics of the 826 Patients According to Sex.*

Characteristic	Women (N=453)	Men (N=373)	P Value
Age — yr	45±18	51±14	<0.001
Site of thrombosis — no. (%)			0.09
Distal veins of the leg	102 (23)	58 (16)	
Proximal veins of the leg	150 (33)	135 (36)	
Axillary veins	19 (4)	14 (4)	
Pulmonary embolism	182 (40)	166 (45)	
Duration of anticoagulation — mo	9±12	8±11	0.76
Follow-up — mo	38±33	33±29	0.02
Factor V Leiden — no. (%)	130 (29)	115 (31)	0.5
Factor II G20210A — no. (%)	36 (8)	25 (7)	0.5
Factor VIII ≥234 IU/dl — no. (%)	44 (10)	28 (8)	0.5
Factor IX ≥138 IU/dl — no. (%)	101 (22)	95 (25)	0.3

* Plus–minus values are means ±SD.

Downloaded from www.nejm.org at OXFORD UNIVERSITY LIBRARY SERVICES on May 8, 2006 .
Copyright © 2004 Massachusetts Medical Society. All rights reserved.

Reproduced with permission from Massachusetts Medical Society.

155

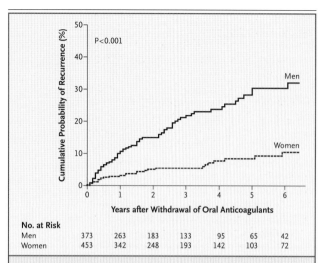

Figure 1. Kaplan–Meier Estimates of the Likelihood of Recurrent Venous Thromboembolism According to Sex.

The cumulative probability of recurrent venous thromboembolism was greater among men than women (P<0.001 by the log-rank test).

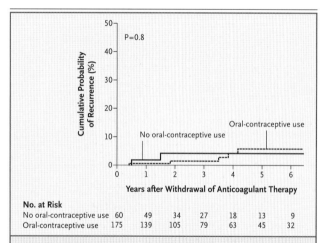

Figure 2. Kaplan–Meier Estimates of the Likelihood of Recurrent Venous Thromboembolism among Women Who Had Their First Venous Thrombosis during Oral-Contraceptive Use, as Compared with Women in the Same Age Group Who Were Not Taking Oral Contraceptives at the Time of a First Thrombotic Event.

The cumulative probability of recurrent venous thromboembolism did not differ significantly between the two groups (P=0.8 by the log-rank test).

replacement therapy had a relative risk of recurrent thromboembolism of 1.6 (95 percent confidence interval, 0.4 to 6.0; P=0.5). In the multivariate analysis, the relative risk of recurrence was 3.4 times as great among men as among women who had not received hormone-replacement therapy (95 percent confidence interval, 2.1 to 5.5; P<0.001).

DISCUSSION

Our study of 826 patients shows that the patient's sex is a major determinant of recurrent venous thromboembolism after an initial episode of spontaneous venous thromboembolism. The risk of recurrence was almost four times as great among men as among women. Five years after the withdrawal of oral anticoagulation, the likelihood of recurrent venous thrombosis was 30.7 percent among men and only 8.5 percent among women (with an upper 95 percent confidence bound of 12.0 percent).

The risk of recurrent venous thrombosis is greatly increased among patients who have had more than one thromboembolic episode[15] and among patients who have cancer,[6] the lupus anticoagulant,[16] or a hereditary deficiency of an inhibitor of coagulation.[17] Patients with these risk factors receive long-term secondary thromboprophylaxis and were therefore not included in our study. Arterial disease or atrial fibrillation developed in a relatively large number of patients during follow-up, and these patients thus began antithrombotic treatment. Given the evidence that oral anticoagulation and aspirin reduce the risk of venous thrombosis and pulmonary embolism,[15,18-20] data on these patients were censored at the time antithrombotic therapy was initiated.

We previously reported that a high level of factor VIII or factor IX or a first symptomatic pulmonary embolism increases the risk of recurrent venous thromboembolism.[21-23] In the current study, however, the proportion of patients with a high level of factor VIII or IX was similar among men and women. In addition, the higher risk of recurrence among men remained unchanged after adjustment for an elevated level of factor VIII or IX and the presence of factor V Leiden, factor II G20210A, and a first symptomatic pulmonary embolism.

Advanced age is an important risk factor for venous thrombosis.[3] The men in our study were on average six years older than the women. The difference in age between the two groups, however, does not explain the higher rate of recurrent venous thromboembolism among men, since the likeli-

Sixty-one women had their first venous thromboembolism during hormone-replacement therapy. As compared with these women, the 108 women in the same age groups who did not use hormone-

Downloaded from www.nejm.org at OXFORD UNIVERSITY LIBRARY SERVICES on May 8, 2006 .
Copyright © 2004 Massachusetts Medical Society. All rights reserved.

Reproduced with permission from Massachusetts Medical Society.

156

hood of recurrence among men and women remained unchanged after adjustment for age.

Oral-contraceptive use increases the risk of venous thrombosis.[24] At the time of their first venous thrombosis, more than a third of the women were taking oral contraceptives, and they were advised to refrain from further oral contraceptive use. These women might have had a lower risk of recurrence — which could explain the low overall risk of recurrence among women — but the risk was low among users and nonusers of oral contraception, and there was no significant difference between the two groups.

Hormone-replacement therapy more than doubles the risk of venous thrombosis.[24] In our study, 61 women had their first thrombotic event while they were taking postmenopausal hormones, but the risk of recurrence among them did not differ significantly from the risk among women who did not use hormone-replacement therapy. Moreover, after these women were excluded from the analysis, the risk of recurrent venous thrombosis was more than three times as great among men as among women in whom the initial episode of thrombosis was not related to postmenopausal hormone use.

Why the women had a low risk of recurrent venous thrombosis is unknown, but the finding may have clinical implications. First, the sex-related difference in the risk of recurrence has to be taken into account in the interpretation of past studies and the design of future trials. Second, the low risk among women could influence decisions concerning the duration of secondary thromboprophylaxis for women, but independent confirmation of our findings is required before they can be translated into routine clinical practice. Third, future studies are warranted to determine whether there are risk factors specific to men or protective factors specific to women.

Supported by grants from the Jubilaeumsfonds of the Österreichische Nationalbank and the Medizinisch-Wissenschaftlicher Fonds des Bürgermeisters der Bundeshauptstadt Wien.

We are indebted to Dr. Marcus Muellner for expert statistical assistance.

REFERENCES

1. Anderson FA Jr, Wheeler HB, Goldberg RJ, et al. A population-based perspective of the hospital incidence and case-fatality rates of deep vein thrombosis and pulmonary embolism: the Worcester DVT Study. Arch Intern Med 1991;151:933-8.
2. Nordstrom M, Lindblad B, Bergqvist D, Kjellstrom T. A prospective study of the incidence of deep-vein thrombosis within a defined urban population. J Intern Med 1992; 232:155-60.
3. White RH. The epidemiology of venous thromboembolism. Circulation 2003;107: Suppl I:I-4–I-8.
4. Oger E. Incidence of venous thromboembolism: a community-based study in western France. Thromb Haemost 2000;83: 657-60.
5. Silverstein MD, Heit JA, Mohr DN, Petterson TM, O'Fallon WM, Melton J III. Trends in the incidence of deep vein thrombosis and pulmonary embolism: a 25-year population-based study. Arch Intern Med 1998;158:585-93.
6. Prandoni P, Lensing AW, Cogo A, et al. The long-term clinical course of acute deep venous thrombosis. Ann Intern Med 1996; 125:1-7.
7. Hansson PO, Sörbo J, Eriksson H. Recurrent venous thromboembolism after deep vein thrombosis: incidence and risk factors. Arch Intern Med 2000;160:769-74.
8. Baglin T, Luddington R, Brown K, Baglin C. Incidence of recurrent venous thromboembolism in relation to clinical and thrombophilic risk factors: prospective cohort study. Lancet 2003;362:523-6.

9. The PIOPED Investigators. Value of the ventilation/perfusion scan in acute pulmonary embolism: results of the Prospective Investigation of Pulmonary Embolism Diagnosis (PIOPED). JAMA 1990;263:2753-69.
10. Bertina RM, Koeleman BP, Koster T, et al. Mutation in blood coagulation factor V associated with resistance to activated protein C. Nature 1994;369:64-7.
11. Poort SR, Rosendaal FR, Reitsma PH, Bertina RM. A common genetic variation in the 3'-untranslated region of the prothrombin gene is associated with elevated plasma prothrombin levels and an increase in venous thrombosis. Blood 1996;88:3698-703.
12. Brandt JT, Triplett DA, Alving B, Scharrer I. Criteria for the diagnosis of lupus anticoagulants: an update. Thromb Haemost 1995;74:1185-90.
13. Kalbfleisch JD, Prentice RL. The statistical analysis of failure time data. New York: John Wiley, 1980.
14. Kaplan EL, Meier P. Nonparametric estimation from incomplete observations. J Am Stat Assoc 1958;53:457-81.
15. Schulman S, Granqvist S, Holmström M, et al. The duration of oral anticoagulant therapy after a second episode of venous thromboembolism. N Engl J Med 1997;336: 393-8.
16. Khamashta MA, Cuadrado MJ, Mujic F, Taub NA, Hunt BJ, Hughes GRV. The management of thrombosis in the antiphospholipid-antibody syndrome. N Engl J Med 1995; 332:993-7.
17. van den Belt AG, Sanson BJ, Simioni P, et al. Recurrence of venous thromboembo-

lism in patients with familial thrombophilia. Arch Intern Med 1997;157:2227-32.
18. Kearon C, Gent M, Hirsh J, et al. A comparison of three months of anticoagulation with extended anticoagulation for a first episode of idiopathic venous thromboembolism. N Engl J Med 1999;340:901-7. [Erratum, N Engl J Med 1999;341:298.]
19. Prevention of pulmonary embolism and deep vein thrombosis with low dose aspirin: Pulmonary Embolism Prevention (PEP) trial. Lancet 2000;355:1295-302.
20. Antiplatelet Trialists' Collaboration. Collaborative overview of randomised trials of antiplatelet therapy. III. Reduction in venous thrombosis and pulmonary embolism by antiplatelet prophylaxis among surgical and medical patients. BMJ 1994;308:235-46.
21. Kyrle PA, Minar E, Hirschl M, et al. High plasma levels of factor VIII and the risk of recurrent venous thromboembolism. N Engl J Med 2000;343:457-62.
22. Weltermann A, Eichinger S, Bialonczyk C, et al. The risk of recurrent venous thromboembolism among patients with high factor IX levels. J Thromb Haemost 2003;1:28-32.
23. Eichinger S, Weltermann A, Minar E, et al. Symptomatic pulmonary embolism and the risk of recurrent venous thromboembolism. Arch Intern Med 2004;164:92-6.
24. Rosendaal FR, van Hylckama Vlieg A, Tanis BC, Helmerhorst FM. Estrogens, progestogens and thrombosis. J Thromb Haemost 2003;1:1371-80.

Copyright © 2004 Massachusetts Medical Society.

Downloaded from www.nejm.org at OXFORD UNIVERSITY LIBRARY SERVICES on May 8, 2006 .
Copyright © 2004 Massachusetts Medical Society. All rights reserved.

Reproduced with permission from Massachusetts Medical Society.

157

Critical appraisal of your own prognostic study

Now use the following sheet to critically appraise an article about prognosis that you have identified in your search sessions.

For your chosen article:

(a) decide whether the internal validity of the study is sufficient to allow firm conclusions (all studies have some flaws; but are these flaws bad enough to discard the study?)

(b) if the study is sufficiently valid, look at and interpret the results — what are the sensitivity, specificity and predictive values for the index test?

Rapid critical appraisal of a prognostic study

Step 1: What question did the study ask?

Population/problem: ....

Indicator: ....

Comparison: ....

Outcome(s): ....

Step 2: How well was the study done? (internal validity)

<table>
<tr><td colspan="2">Recruitment — Was a defined representative sample of patients assembled at a common (usually early) point in the course of their disease?</td></tr>
<tr><td>What is best?</td><td>Where do I find the information?</td></tr>
<tr><td>Patients should ideally be enrolled at a uniformly early time in the disease; called an 'inception cohort'. Patients should also be representative of the underlying population. Patients from tertiary referral centres may have more advanced disease and poorer prognoses than patients from primary care.</td><td>The Methods section should describe the stage at which patients entered the study (eg at the time of first myocardial infarction; Stage 3 breast cancer). The Methods section should also provide information about patient recruitment, including whether patients were recruited from primary care or tertiary referral centres.</td></tr>
<tr><td colspan="2">This paper:　Yes ☐　No ☐　Unclear ☐　Comment: ....</td></tr>
<tr><td colspan="2">Adjustment — How were patients treated? If subgroups with different prognoses are identified, did adjustment for important prognostic factors take place?</td></tr>
<tr><td>What is best?</td><td>Where do I find the information?</td></tr>
<tr><td>The study should report how patients were treated, and adjust or stratify results by treatment. For new prognostic factors — a patient characteristic (eg age, stage of disease) that predicts the patient's eventual outcome — the study should adjust for known prognostic factors in the analysis so that the results indicate the additional prognostic information.</td><td>The Results section should identify any treatments and prognostic factors and whether these have been adjusted for in the analysis. Also look at the tables and figures (eg there may be separate survival curves for patients at different stages of disease or for different age groups).</td></tr>
<tr><td colspan="2">This paper:　Yes ☐　No ☐　Unclear ☐　Comment: ....</td></tr>
</table>

*M*aintenance — Was the comparable status of the study groups maintained through equal management?	
What is best?	**Where do I find the information?**
Prognosis is always conditional on treatment, and hence initial and subsequent treatment should be clearly spelt out, and an assessment given on the likely impact of this treatment on the 'natural history' (the course of illness without treatment).	Look in the **Methods** section for information on the management of the study groups during the follow-up period (such as follow-up schedule, permitted additional activities or exposures) and in **Results** for any further information.

This paper: Yes ☐   No ☐   Unclear ☐   Comment: ....

.... and adequate follow-up?

What is best?	**Where do I find the information?**
Follow-up should be long enough to detect the outcome of interest (eg for pregnancy outcomes, nine months; for cancer, many years). All patients should be followed until the outcomes of interest or death occurs. Reasons for loss to follow-up should be provided, along with the characteristics of those patients.	The **Results** section should say how many subjects were allocated to each group (eg baseline characteristics table) and how many were actually included in the analysis. You will need to read the results section to clarify the number of and reason for losses to follow-up.

This paper: Yes ☐   No ☐   Unclear ☐   Comment: ....

*M*easurement — Were the subjects and assessors kept 'blind' to which treatment was being received and/or were the measures objective?	
What is best?	**Where do I find the information?**
It is ideal if both the outcome assessors and the subjects are blinded to the nature of the study groups. If the outcome is objective (eg death) then blinding is less critical. If the outcome is subjective (eg symptoms or function) then blinding of the outcome assessor is critical.	The **Methods** section should describe how the outcome was assessed and whether the assessor/s were aware of the subjects' groups.

This paper: Yes ☐   No ☐   Unclear ☐   Comment: ....

Step 3: What do the results mean?

What measure was used and how large was the treatment effect?	
Could the effect have been due to chance?	
P-value	
Confidence interval (CI)	

Critical appraisal of studies for a diagnostic test accuracy question

In EBP Step 1 (Formulate an answerable question) we saw how the PICO method of formulating a health care question can be used for questions about the accuracy of diagnostic tests (population/problem, index test, control, outcome). We also noted that the ideal type of study to answer this type of question — see the levels of evidence table — is a 'cross-sectional study with a random or consecutive sample' (see page 42).

A cross-sectional study examines health-related characteristics in patients at a single time point — that is, the I and O are measured at the same time. The aim of a cross-sectional diagnostic study is to find out how well the new (or index) test identifies those people with or without the condition (outcome) in patients with a particular clinical presentation (P). In order to do this, it is necessary for each subject in the study to have two independent tests or assessments:

▶ the test under consideration (index test)

▶ another test or investigation that will show whether the condition is present or not (the reference standard or 'gold' standard).

The reference standard may be:

▶ a different test that is known to give an accurate answer (but that may be more expensive or more invasive than the new test)

▶ a composite of several tests

▶ the result of another medical procedure (such as surgery)

▶ the outcome of a period of follow-up (indicating whether the person develops the condition in question).

So, if your question was about diagnosis and you have found a diagnostic cross-sectional study, how would you know if the results are reliable? Again, we turn to critical appraisal using the same principles that we have already discussed for RCTs:

▶ Question 1: How well does the PICO of the study match your PICO?

▶ Question 2: How well was the study done (RAMMbo)?

▶ Question 3: What do the results mean?

We will not walk you through a paper this time, but ask you to go straight ahead and try appraising one yourself using the boxes provided below. Some suggested 'answers' are in the 'Answers' section in Part 4 of this workbook. To set the scene, imagine you have read a recent review in the *Journal of the American Medical Association* suggesting the whispered voice test is the best way to screen for hearing deficits, but you want to look at one of the papers this is based on to double check the validity and also to learn how they did the test.

In other words, your clinical question is:

P   *In people with possible hearing problems…*

I/C   *… is the whispered voice test accurate (ie how sensitive and specific is it) …*

O   *… for diagnosing true hearing deficits?*

After searching in PubMed, imagine that you find the following paper:

> Eekhof JA, de Bock GH, de Laat JAPM, Dap R, Schaapveld K, Springer MP (1996). The whispered voice: The best test for screening hearing for impairment in general practice? *British Journal of General Practice* 46:473–474. (The full article is included on pages 169–170 of this workbook.)

Question 1: How well does the PICO of the study match your PICO?

As for the RCT example, it is a good idea to work out what the PICO of the paper is to find out whether it matches your original PICO.

What is the PICO of the whispered voice test study?

Question 2: How well was the study done?

The approach to critically appraising articles on diagnostic tests is similar to that for RCTs. The main difference is that instead of having two groups with random allocation, the subjects all receive both the index test and the reference standard. For an accuracy study, that's all you need.

(Note: If you want to assess the impact on the subjects of having or not having the test then you might need a randomised trial, but not for simply estimating accuracy. Accuracy will be important but the impact also depends on many other factors, including other tests and subsequent treatments.)

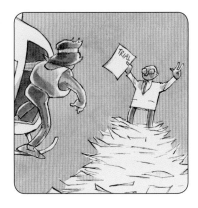

RAMMbo to the rescue

Recruitment

The subjects should be representative of the folk with the problem that the test is aimed at. (Ideally, they should include a spectrum of cases with respect to both severity and timing of symptoms.)

> **Recruitment — How were the participants in the whispered voice test study recruited?**
>
> ....
>
> ....
>
> ....

Allocation

For studies of diagnostic accuracy, there is no allocation to groups. All subjects should receive the index test and the reference standard. The relevant aspect of 'allocation', in this case, is that both the test and the standard should be applied independently to all the subjects.

> **Allocation — How were the index and reference standard applied in the whispered voice test study?**
>
> ....
>
> ....
>
> ....

Maintenance

All the recruited patients should be maintained in the study (that is, they should receive both the index and reference test).

> **Maintenance — How were the participants in the whispered voice test study managed?**
>
> ....
>
> ....
>
> ....

Measurement

The results should be measured EITHER with everyone
blinded to the results of the index test, OR with an
objective test endpoint (such as death or a laboratory machine that can't be bribed or biased).

> **Measurement — How were the outcomes measured in the whispered voice test study?**
>
> ....
>
> ....
>
> ....

Question 3: What do the results mean?

There are two types of results commonly reported in diagnostic test studies. The first concerns the accuracy of the test and is reflected in two measures:

▶   sensitivity (how often we get positive results in folk with the condition)

▶   specificity (how often we get negative results in folk without the condition).

Ideally, these measures should both be 100% but they rarely are! More often there will be some false positives and some false negatives. If they are both 50% (or together add up to 100%) then the test is useless, because it is equivalent to a coin toss.

The second concerns how the test performs in the population being tested and is reflected in the post-test probabilities (also called predictive values):

▶   post-test probability after a positive test (also called the positive predictive value): the proportion of people with a positive test who have the condition

▶   post-test probability after a negative test (the negative predictive value): the proportion of people with a negative test who do not have the condition.

As an example, consider the MiniCog test (a clockface drawing plus 3-item recall) for a quick test for dementia.

The results in a community sample are shown in the table below.

		Reference standard		
		+ve	-ve	Total
Index test	+ve	58	115	173
	-ve	18	928	946
	Total	76	1043	1119

Reference:

Borson S, Scanlan JM, Chen P, Ganquli M (2003). The Mini-Cog as a screen for dementia: validation in a population-based sample. *Journal of the American Geriatric Society* 51:1451–1454.

From this we can calculate the following values:

Measure	Meaning
Sensitivity (Sn) = the proportion of people with the condition who have a positive test result In our example, the Sn = 58/76 = 0.76 (76%)	The sensitivity tells us how well the test identifies people with the condition. A highly sensitive test will not miss many people.
False negative rate (1-sensitivity)	Only 18/1119 people (1.6%) with dementia were falsely identified as not having it. This means the test is fairly good at identifying people with the condition.
Specificity (Sp) = the proportion of people without the condition who have a negative test result In our example, the Sp = 928/1043 = 0.86 (86%)	The specificity tells us how well the test identifies people without the condition. A highly specific test will not falsely identify many people as having the condition.
False positive rate (1-specificity)	However, 115/1119 people (10%) without dementia were falsely identified as having it. This means the test is only moderately good at identifying people without the condition.
Positive predictive value (PPV) = the proportion of people with a positive test who have the condition	This measure tells us how well the test performs in this population. It is dependent on the accuracy of the test (primarily specificity) and the prevalence of the condition.
In our example, the PPV = 58/173 = 0.33 (33%)	Of the 173 people who had a positive test result, 33% will actually have dementia.
Negative predictive value (NPV) = the proportion of people with a negative test who do not have the condition	This measure tells us how well the test performs in this population. It is dependent on the accuracy of the test and the prevalence of the condition.
In our example, the NPV = 928/946 = 0.98 (98%)	Of the 946 people who had a negative test result, 98% will not have dementia.

To further explore the meaning of all these terms, consider a situation in which 1000 elderly people with suspected dementia undergo an index test and a reference standard. Suppose the prevalence of dementia in this group is 25%, compared with the 7% in the study we looked at above (76/1119). Of the group, 240 people tested positive on both the index test and the reference standard, and 600 people tested negative on both tests.

The first step is to draw a 2 x 2 table as shown below. We are told that the prevalence of dementia is 25%; therefore, we can fill in the last row of totals — 25% of 1000 people is 250 people — so 250 people will have dementia and 750 people will be free from dementia. This is the bottom row of the table. Next we can work out the split of those with disease from the sensitivity. 76% of the 250 people (that is, 190 people) will be positive. By subtraction, the other 60 people must be index test negative.

Reference standard

		+ve	-ve	Total
Index test	+ve	190		
	-ve	60		
	Total	250	750	1000

We can now repeat the process with the non-demented column of 750 people. Of these, 89% will be MiniCog negative (that is, 668 people). And by subtraction, 82 people must be negative:

Reference standard

		+ve	-ve	Total
Index test	+ve	190	82	272
	-ve	60	668	728
	Total	250	750	1000

Now we are ready to re-calculate the post-test probabilities in the different population. Working across the rows we can see that:

▶ post-test probability after a positive = 190/272 = 0.69 (69%) and

▶ post-test probability after a negative = 60/728 = 0.08 (8%).

So notice that the post-test probabilities are different in this higher-prevalence population where we suspected dementia. We have assumed that the sensitivity and specificity have remained constant. While this is not always exactly true, it is a reasonable approximation. To find out more on methods for calculating post-test probabilities, see the article by Paul Glasziou ('Which methods for bedside Bayes?') in the 'Further reading' section in Part 4 of this workbook.

Now try to answer the following questions for the whispered voice test (answers are in the 'Answers' section in Part 4 of this workbook).

What do the results of the whispered voice test study mean?

1. Fill in the following 2x2 table and then calculate the values below:

Reference standard (ENT audiometer)

	+ve	-ve	Total
Index test (whispered voice test) +ve			
-ve			
Total			

Sensitivity (Sn): ....

Specificity (SP): ....

Post-test probability after a positive: ....

Post-test probability after a negative: ....

2. How did the whispered voice test compare to other tests reported in the paper?

....

....

Summary of critical appraisal of the whispered voice test

R ....

A ....

M ....

M **b** **o** ....

Results ....

....

Overall ....

....

The whispered voice: The best test for screening for hearing impairment in general practice?

JUST A H EEKHOF

GEERTRUIDA H de BOCK

JAN A P M de LAAT

RAYMOND DAP

KEES SCHAAPVELD

MACHIEL P SPRINGER

SUMMARY

Hearing loss is an important health problem in the elderly which sometimes leads to social isolation. In a study with 62 patients, the diagnostic value of four simple tests for screening for hearing loss in general practice was examined. When paying attention to the loudness of the whispering, the whispered voice test can be a valuable test for assessment of hearing loss in general practice.

Keywords: hearing loss; elderly patients; whispered voice test.

Introduction

Hearing loss of 35 dB and over is a common health problem in the elderly that can lead to social isolation. In the UK, general practitioners have been obliged to screen the elderly for hearing loss since the 1990 National Health Service contract. While its diagnostic value is still in debate, the Royal College of General Practitioners has chosen the whispered voice as the first test for hearing loss.[1] In the Netherlands, general practitioners also need a simple method to identify elderly people with hearing loss. The principal aim of this study was to investigate the diagnostic value of the whispered voice test.

Method

The diagnostic value of the whispered voice test was investigated (1) by comparing its sensitivity and specificity to other simple diagnostic tests, using the audiogram as a reference standard, and (2) by examining the interobserver reliability of the whispered voice.[2] The results of six other examiners with the whispered voice were compared with the results of the first examiner and expressed by means of sensitivity/specificity and Cohen's

J A H Eekhof, MD, general practitioner, Department of General Practice, Leiden University; G H De Bock, PhD, psychologist and epidemiologist, Department of General Practice and Medical Decision Making Unit, Leiden University; J A P M De Laat, PhD, physicist and audiologist, Audiological Centre, Ear, Nose and Throat Department, University Hospital Leiden; R Dap, medical student, Department of General Practice, Leiden University; K Schaapveld, MD, PhD, public health scientist, TNO Prevention and Health, Leiden; and M P Springer, MD, PhD, professor of general practice, Department of General Practice, Leiden University, Leiden, the Netherlands.
Submitted: 24 July 1995; accepted: 18 March 1996.

© *British Journal of General Practice*, 1996, **46,** 473-474.

Kappa.

In a period of 6 weeks, all patients aged 55 years and over, attending an outpatient ENT department for an audiogram were studied. Patients using a hearing aid were excluded. The tests were performed in a consulting room where the amount of extraneous noise was comparable to general practice.

The pure-tone thresholds of the reference test were assessed with an ENT audiometer using a standard method.[3] Because we performed the four tests in the way they were originally validated, the four tests had different screening levels. Therefore, we compared the results with the same level at the reference test:

(1) The whispered voice was performed by a standard method (slightly modified).[4] Inability to repeat two or more combinations correctly was regarded as a hearing loss of more than 30 dB. The test was performed for a second time by six other examiners.

(2) The Pat-225 involves pushing a button to produce a mixed noise (from approximately 500 to 4000 Hz) of 30 dB, and its has to be held 25 cm from the test ear. The test was positive when the noise was heard.

(3) The Audioscope-3 is an auroscope with a built-in audiometric screening device.[5] Patients who did not hear all four tones were considered to have a hearing loss of more than 40 dB.

(4) A screening audiometer (Micromate-304) was limited to use at 2000 and 4000 Hz at 40 dB, which can be performed within 3 min. Patients passed if they could hear both tones.

Results

Out of 62 patients, 124 ears were studied. Because there was only a low correlation between the results of the two ears of the same subject (Pearson's R 0.18), we treated the ears as independent.

According to the reference test of the ENT audiometer, 73 out of the 124 ears had a hearing loss of >30 dB and 41 had a hearing loss of >40 dB.

According to the whispered voice test, 76 ears had a hearing loss of >30 dB: sensitivity and specificity were 90% (66/73, 95% CI 84–97) and 80% (41/51, 95% CI 69–91). With the Madsen Pat 225, 88 ears had a hearing loss of >30 dB: the sensitivity and specificity of this test were 88% (64/73, 95% 80–95) and 53% (27/51, 95% CI 39–66). With the Audioscope-3, 89 ears had a hearing loss of >40 dB: the sensitivity and specificity were 100% (41/41) and 42% (35/83, 95% CI 32–57). Using the screening audiometer, 92 ears had a hearing loss of >40 dB: sensitivity and specificity were 100% (41/41) and 39% (32/83, 95% CI 28–49).

Among the six other examiners with the whispered voice, the sensitivity varied from 93 to 100%, the specificity from 14 to 100% and Cohen's kappa from 0.16 to 1.0 (Table 1).

Discussion

The whispered voice is the best among the available simple tests to identify people with hearing loss in general practice with respect to sensitivity and specificity. However, there was a broad

Reproduced with permission from *British Journal of General Practice*.

J A H Eekhof, G H De Bock, J A M De Laat, *et al*

Table 1. Sensitivity and specificity of the whispered voice test by examiners 2 to 7, and the inter-observer reliability when compared with examiner 1 (Cohen's Kappa).

	Examiner					
	2	3	4	5	6	7
Ears <30 dB (*n*/total)	1/32	16/24	19/36	11/16	8/12	3/4
Sensitivity/ specificity	100/29	93/56	100/42	100/14	100/80	100/100
Examiner 1** (Kappa)	0.31	0.52	0.42	0.16	0.82	1.0

*With the reference test. **Examiner 1: sensitivity, 80; specificity, 80; *n* = 124.

variation between outcomes of the examiners. A possible explanation is the difference in loudness of the whispering. It might be that examiners 6 and 7 whispered too loudly, indicated by a low sensitivity and a high specificity. However, because examiners 2 to 5 all had a high sensitivity and a low specificity, we assume that they all whispered too quietly. This conclusion is supported by some patients who spontaneously complained about the very quiet whispering of examiners 2 and 5. While performing the whispered voice test, one should pay attention to the loudness of the whispering.

In the RCGP guidelines for the annual screening of the elderly for assessing hearing loss, the choice was made in favour of the whispered voice on pragmatic grounds.[1] Although we had a small sample size, we can draw the conclusion that the whispered voice is an appropriate test to objectify hearing loss in general practice, especially when we included the purchasing costs of the different tests (whispered voice = 0, Madsen Pat-225 = £83, Welch-Allyn Audioscope-3 = £491 and Madsen Micromate-304 = £893). Taking these limitations into account, the whispered voice can be a valuable test for assessment of hearing loss by the general practitioner.

References

1. Williams EI, Wallace P. *Health checks for people aged 75 and over* [Occasional paper 59]. London: Royal College of General Practitioners, 1993.
2. Lichenstein MJ, Bess FH, Logan SA. Screening for impaired hearing in the elderly [reply to a letter to the editor]. *JAMA* 1988; **260:** 3589–3589.
3. British Society of Audiology. Recommended procedures for pure-tone audiometry. *Br J Audiol* 1983; **15:** 213–216.
4. Swan IRC, Browning GG. The whispered voice as a screening test for hearing impairment. *J Roy Coll Gen Practitioners* 1985; **35:** 197.
5. Lichenstein MJ, Bess FH, Logan SA. Validation of screening tools for identifying hearing-impaired elderly in primary care. *JAMA* 1988; **259:** 2875–2878.

Address for correspondence
JAH Eekhof, Department of General Practice, Leiden University, PO Box 2088, 2301 CB Leiden, the Netherlands.

Reproduced with permission from *British Journal of General Practice.*

Critical appraisal of your own diagnostic test accuracy study

Use the following sheet to critically appraise an article about a diagnostic test that you have identified in one of your search sessions.

For your chosen article:

(a) decide whether the internal validity of the study is sufficient to allow firm conclusions (all studies have some flaws; but are these flaws bad enough to discard the study?)

(b) if the study is sufficiently valid, look at and interpret the results — what are the sensitivity, specificity and predictive values for the index test?

Rapid critical appraisal of a diagnostic test accuracy study

Step 1: What question did the study ask?

Population/problem: ....

Index case: ....

Comparison: ....

Outcome(s): ....

Step 2: How well was the study done? (internal validity)

Recruitment — Was the diagnostic test evaluated in a representative spectrum of patients (like those in whom it would be used in practice)?	
What is best?	**Where do I find the information?**
It is ideal if the diagnostic test is applied to the full spectrum of patients — those with mild, severe, early and late cases of the target disorder. It is also best if the patients are randomly selected or consecutive admissions so that selection bias is minimised.	The **Methods** section should tell you how patients were enrolled and whether they were randomly selected or consecutive admissions. It should also tell you where patients came from and whether they are likely to be representative of the patients in whom the test is to be used.
This paper: Yes ☐ No ☐ Unclear ☐ Comment:	

Maintenance — Was the endpoint of the reference standard obtained for all the subjects?	
What is best?	**Where do I find the information?**
The endpoint of the reference standard (ie whether the subjects are positive or negative for the condition) should be measured for all the subjects. In cases where this depends on the follow-up of people for a period of time (dependent on the disease in question) to see whether they are truly negative, this follow-up should be long enough to be certain of the outcome.	The **Methods** section should indicate whether the endpoint of the reference standard was obtained for all subjects.
This paper: Yes ☐ No ☐ Unclear ☐ Comment:	

Measurement — Were the assessors kept **b**lind to the results of each test and/or were the reference standard endpoints **O**bjective?	
What is best?	**Where do I find the information?**
The reference standard and the index test being assessed should be applied to each patient independently and blindly. Those who interpreted the results of one test should not be aware of the results of the other test. Finally, the paper should also have sufficient description of the index test to allow its replication and also interpretation of the results.	The **Methods** section should describe who conducted the two tests and whether each was conducted independently and blinded to the results of the other. The **Methods** section should describe the tests in detail.

This paper: Yes ☐ No ☐ Unclear ☐ Comment: ....

Step 3: What do the results mean?

Reference standard

Measure	Result
Sensitivity (Sn)	
Specificity (Sp)	
Positive predictive value (PPV)	
Negative predictive value (NPV)	

Notes

Part 4

Reflections and further information

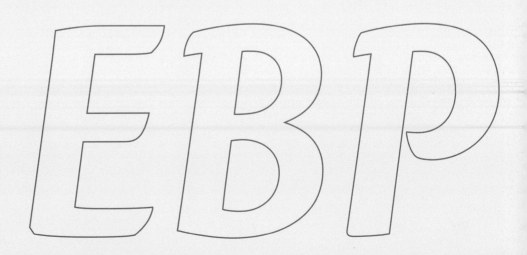

How am I doing?
Diary of a reflective practitioner

Evaluating the effectiveness of your EBP process is sometimes suggested as Step 5 of the EBP process, but it is really a 'meta-step' which asks how you are doing at the other 4 steps. It is important to keep records of your clinical questions, research results and critical appraisal of evidence, to follow up patients for whom you have applied the results of your searches and to record and, where appropriate, publish the outcomes. This clinical audit of your EBP activities will help you to improve what you are doing and to share your findings with clinical colleagues. Some of the questions you may need to include in your self-audit are discussed below.

Are you asking any questions at all?

Ask yourself if you have managed to find the time and motivation to write down your information needs as they arise in a way that you can follow up to a clinically useful conclusion.

If not, you may be missing some opportunities to improve your clinical knowledge and performance. You could revisit the section on formulating answerable questions (EBP Step 1) and look for other strategies, such as teaming up with some colleagues to take this on as a group. You could also try asking your colleagues 'What is the evidence for that?' whenever they make a pronouncement on the most appropriate management approach to a clinical problem.

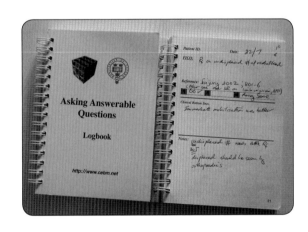

Whatever else you do we suggest one crucial step is to have a question logbook (see picture at right) to keep a record of your questions and answers. This will allow you to keep track of questions and see how many you are answering, and will provide a permanent record so you can look up old answers later when you need them.

Write your reflections here:

What is your success rate in asking answerable questions?

If you are generating questions, you need to ask whether your success rate in framing answerable questions is rising. If you have a questions logbook this will enable you to do a simple count and to see what sort of questions you ask. If your success rate is high enough for you to keep asking questions, all is well. If you are becoming discouraged, however, you could talk to your colleagues who are having greater success and try to learn from them or attend some further professional development workshops on EBM.

> **Write your reflections here:**
>
> ....
>
> ....
>
> ....
>
> ....

How is your searching going?

If you are generating and framing answerable questions, you need to ask if you are following them up with searches and whether you have teady access to the necessary searching tools: the computers, internet access, software and the best evidence for your discipline. You could also run an audit of your questions against the resources that you found most useful for finding answers.

Other questions you might like to ask yourself include:

▶ Do you have the best evidence readily available in your clinical working area?

▶ Are you finding useful evidence from a widening array of sources?

▶ Are you becoming more efficient in your searching?

▶ Are you using MeSH headings?

▶ How do your searches compare to those of research librarians or other respected colleagues?

If you are having trouble with the effectiveness of your searching, you could consult your nearest health library for further information on how to access and use the available search engines and other resources. You might also want to check and reduce any barriers to searching. Are your best evidence resources bookmarked and readily available in the browser in your consulting room? Perhaps you could make your favourite resource your homepage. Do you need to subscribe to any other resources?

Write your reflections here:

JUST CHECKING ALL THE EVIDENCE

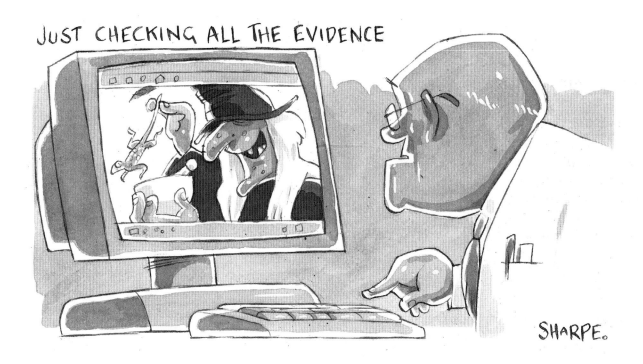

SHARPE.

Are you critically appraising your search results?

First, you should ask yourself whether you are critically appraising your evidence at all. If so, are you becoming more efficient and accurate at applying critical appraisal guidelines and measures (such as NNTs)? You may be able to find this out by comparing your results with those of colleagues who are appraising the same evidence. Of course, you will be slow at first but, with practice, it is possible to do appraisals in 5–10 minutes (and really flawed studies can often be tossed away in seconds).

Write your reflections here:

Are you applying your evidence in clinical practice?

You need to ask yourself if you are integrating your critical appraisals with your clinical expertise and applying the results in your clinical practice. If so, are you becoming more accurate and efficient in adjusting some of the critical appraisal measures to fit your individual patients?

A good way to test your skills in this integration is to see whether you can use them to explain (and, hopefully, resolve) disputes about management decisions.

Write your reflections here:

Are you sharing your efforts with others?

Finally, you should ask about how well you are working with others on improvement. Working with others in the clinical team makes this more fun, and also serves to share the effort and as a checkpoint on your interpretations. We strongly encourage some group activity with your EBP. If you work solo you might join an email discussion list. So ask yourself:

▶ Do you have a regular clinical discussion session where you look at evidence (a 'journal club')?

▶ Do you have a means of sharing search and appraisal results (a book or intranet)?

▶ How could you improve the team processes (best to discuss this with the team!)?

Reference:

Sackett DL, Straus SE, Richardson WS, Rosenberg W, Haynes RB (2000). *Evidence-Based Medicine. How to Practice and Teach EBM* (2nd edition), Churchill Livingstone, Edinburgh.

Write your reflections here:

Notes

Useful sources of evidence

Studies

PubMed Clinical Queries

http://www.ncbi.nlm.nih.gov/entrez/query/static/clinical.html

PubMed is a free internet MEDLINE database. The Clinical Queries section is a question-focused interface with filters for identifying the more appropriate studies for questions of therapy, prognosis, diagnosis and etiology.

SUMSearch

http://sumsearch.uthscsa.edu

A super-PubMed: SUMSearch simultaneously searches multiple internet sites and collates the results. Checks for the Merck manual, guidelines, systematic reviews and PubMed Clinical Queries entries.

Cochrane Library and Collaboration

http://www.cochrane.org

The Cochrane Library is the single best source of reliable evidence about the effects of health care. The Cochrane Trials Registry contains over 300,000 controlled trials – the best single repository.

CINAHL

http://www.cinahl.com/

CINAHL is the Cumulative Index to Nursing and Allied Health Literature. Unlike PubMed Clinical Queries, it has no inbuilt filters.

Appraised studies

Evidence-Based Medicine

http://www.evidence-basedmedicine.com

A bimonthly journal which summarises important recent articles from major clinical fields (family medicine, internal medicine, obstetrics and gynecology, pediatrics, psychiatry, public health, surgery). (Note: The cumulated contents of *Evidence-Based Medicine* (since 1995) and *ACP Journal Club*, which is a publication of the American College of Physicians (since 1991), are published annually on a CD called Best Evidence.

PEDro

http://www.pedro.fhs.usyd.edu.au/

A physiotherapy trials database with over 2300 controlled trials, many of which have been appraised by the PEDro team.

OTseeker

http://www.otseeker.com/

OTseeker is a database that contains abstracts of systematic reviews and randomised controlled trials relevant to occupational therapy.

BestBETS

http://www.bestbets.org

Provides rapid evidence-based answers to real-life clinical questions in emergency medicine, using a systematic approach to reviewing the literature. BETs take into account the shortcomings of much current evidence, allowing physicians to make the best of what there is. Developed in the Emergency Department of Manchester Royal Infirmary, UK.

Syntheses

Cochrane Library and Collaboration

http://www.cochrane.org

The Cochrane Database of Systematic Reviews has over 1000 systematic reviews done by The Cochrane Collaboration. The Database of Abstracts of Reviews of Effectiveness (DARE) database lists other systematic reviews.

Synopses

Clinical Evidence

http://www.clinicalevidence.com

Clinical Evidence is an updated directory of evidence on the effects of clinical interventions. It summarises the current state of knowledge, ignorance, and uncertainty about the prevention and treatment of clinical conditions, based on thorough searches and appraisal of the literature. It covers 20 specialties and includes 134 conditions. Updated/expanded coverage every six months in print and on CD.

Bandolier

http://www.jr2.ox.ac.uk/bandolier/index.html

A monthly newsletter of evidence distributed in the NHS, which is freely downloadable.

TRIP Database

http://www.tripdatabase.com

Searches several different evidence-based resources including PubMed, Bandolier, and the ATTRACT question-answering service. Only allows title searches, but does allow AND, OR, NOT

Further reading

The steps of EBP

Haynes RB (2001). Of studies, syntheses, synopses, and systems: the "4S" evolution of services for finding current best evidence. *ACP Journal Club* 134(2): A11–13.

Jackson R, Ameratunga S, Broad J, Connor J et al (2006). The GATE frame: Critical appraisal with pictures. *ACP Journal Club* 144(2):A8–11.

Edwards A, Elwyn G, Mulley A (2002). Explaining risks: turning numerical data into meaningful pictures. *British Medical Journal* 324(7341):827–830.

Glasziou P (2001). Which methods for bedside Bayes? *ACP Journal Club* 135: A11–12.

Statistics

Carney S, Doll H (2005). Introduction to biostatistics: Part 1. Measurement scales and their summary statistics. *ACP Journal Club* 143(1):A8–9.

Carney S, Doll H (2005). Introduction to biostatistics: Part 2. Measures of association as used to address therapy, harm, and etiology questions. *ACP Journal Club* 143:A8.

Carney S, Doll H (2005). Statistical approaches to uncertainty: *P* values and confidence intervals unpacked. *Evidence-Based Medicine* 10:133–134.

Glasziou P, Doll H (2006). Was the study big enough? Two café rules. *Evidence-Based Medicine* 11:69–70.

EBP in practice: examples and issues

Phillips RS, Glasziou P (2004). What makes evidence-based journal clubs succeed? *ACP Journal Club* 140(3):A11–12.

Glasziou P, Haynes B (2005). The paths from research to improved health outcomes. *ACP Journal Club* 142(2):A8–10.

Glasziou P (2004). Practice corner: the first symptom of hyperkalemia is death. *ACP Journal Club* 140(2):A13.

Heneghan C (2005). Practice corner: The doctor's advice and sleepless nights: what can you find in 5 minutes? *Evidence-Based Medicine* 10:36–38.

Glossary

Absolute risk reduction

The difference between the rate of relevant outcomes in the treatment and control groups.

Accuracy (*see also* **Diagnostic accuracy**)

The degree to which a measurement represents the true value of the variable measured.

Adjustment (*see also* **Confounding**)

A procedure for minimising differences in the composition of populations being compared using statistical methods.

Allocation

The way that subjects are assigned to the different groups in a study (eg drug treatment vs placebo; usual treatment vs no treatment).

All-or-none evidence

Is when all patients died before the treatment became available, but some now survive on it; or when some patients died before the treatment became available, but none now die on it. For a refinement of this see: Glasziou P, et al (2007). When are randomised trials unnecessary? Picking signal from noise. *British Medical Journal* 334:349–51.

Applicability (*see also* **External validity**)

Addresses whether a particular treatment or exposure that showed an overall effect in a study can be expected to convey the same effect for an individual or group in a specific clinical or population setting.

Bias

Deviation of a measurement from the 'true' value leading to either an over- or underestimation of the treatment effect. Bias can originate from many different sources, such as allocation of patients, measurement, interpretation, publication and review of data.

Blinding

A study protocol that prevents those involved in a clinical study from knowing to which treatment groups subjects have been assigned. Blinding of the subjects themselves minimises bias in patient responses; blinding of outcome assessors minimises biasing in measurements.

Case-control study

A study in which a group of patients with a specific outcome are matched with a group of matched controls without the outcome and information is obtained about their past exposure to a factor under investigation.

Glossary adapted from *How to Review the Evidence: Systematic Identification and Review of the Scientific Literature*, National Health and Medical Research Council, Canberra, Australia, 2000.

Case series

Outcome information collected for a series (consecutive or non-consecutive) of patients after a treatment or exposure (ie with no control group). For a pre-test/post-test case series, measures are taken before and after the intervention is introduced to a series of people and are then compared (also known as a 'before-and-after study').

Cohort study

A study in which data are obtained from matched groups who have been either exposed or not exposed (controls) to a new technology, prognostic factor or risk factor. There are two study designs:

- prospective — the cohorts are identified at a point in time (such as time of birth, residence at a specific location, exposure to a particular risk factor) and followed forward in time to record health outcomes

- retrospective — the cohorts are defined at a point of time in the past and information is collected on subsequent outcomes.

An 'inception cohort' is a group of patients assembled near the onset of the target disorder (such as at the time of first exposure to a supposed cause) and followed forward in time.

Comparator

Treatment, prognostic indicator or test that is compared with the treatment, indicator or test of interest in a clinical trial.

Confidence interval (CI)

An interval within which the population parameter (the 'true' value) is expected to lie with a given degree of certainty (eg 95%).

Confounding (*see also* **Adjustment**)

The distortion of the true effect of treatment (or a risk factor) by other factors that vary between the study and control groups (eg baseline differences in age, sex or lifestyle).

Critical appraisal

Process of assessing how well the methods of a clinical study eliminate bias (and therefore how reliable the results are). Process of (a) assessing how well the methods of a clinical study eliminate bias and therefore how reliable the results are (which is also called 'internal validity'); and (b) interpreting what the results mean.

Cross-sectional study

A study that examines the relationship between specific outcomes and variables of interest in a defined population at a particular time (ie exposure and outcomes are both measured at the same time). For a diagnostic cross-sectional study, a consecutive group of subjects receive both the test under study (index test) and the reference standard test.

Diagnostic case-control study (*see also* **Case–control study**)

A study in which the index test results for a group of patients already known to have the disease (through the reference standard) are compared to the index test results for a separate group of normal/healthy people known to be free of the disease (through the reference standard).

Diagnostic accuracy

A measure of how often a diagnostic test gives the right answer (that is, positive result for people with the condition and negative result for people without it).

Evidence-based practice (also called evidence-based medicine)

Patient care in which clinical expertise and patient values are integrated with the best research evidence from the medical literature.

Experimental studies

Studies in which subjects are allocated to two or more groups to receive an intervention, exposure or test and then followed up under carefully controlled conditions.

External validity (*see also* **Applicability, Validity**)

The degree to which the results of a clinical study can be applied to clinical practice in a specific setting.

Hazard ratio (HR)

The ratio of the hazards in the treatment and control groups where the hazard is the probability of having the outcome at time t, given that the outcome has not occurred up to time t.

Heterogeneity

Differences in treatment effect between studies contributing to a meta-analysis. Significant heterogeneity suggests that the trials are not estimating a single common treatment effect.

Index test (*see also* **Reference test**)

In a diagnostic study, the index test is the test for which the diagnostic accuracy is being measured.

Intention to treat

Analysis of clinical trial participants according to the group to which they were initially allocated, regardless of whether or not they dropped out, fully complied with the treatment, or crossed over to the other treatment.

Interrupted time series (*see* **Time series**)

Intervention

A therapeutic procedure, such as treatment with a pharmaceutical agent, surgery, a dietary supplement, a dietary change, psychotherapy, early detection (screening) or use of patient educational materials.

Level of evidence

A hierarchy of study designs according to their internal validity, or degree to which they are not susceptible to bias.

Meta-analysis

Results from several studies, identified in a systematic review, are combined and summarised quantitatively.

Null hypothesis

Presumption that the results observed in a study (eg the apparent beneficial effects of an intervention) were due to chance.

Number needed to treat (NNT)

The number of patients with a particular condition who must receive a treatment in order to prevent the occurrence of one adverse outcome. NNT is the inverse of the absolute risk reduction. Similarly, 'number needed to harm' (NNH) refers to harmful outcomes.

Odds ratio (OR)

Ratio of the odds (those with the outcome divided by those without it) in the treatment group to the corresponding odds in the control group. An odds ratio of 1 implies that the outcome is equally likely in both groups.

Primary research

Individual studies such as a randomised controlled trial, cohort study etc.

Prognostic indicator

A factor (such as age, gender, risk factor) that is related to a person's probability of developing the disease or outcome.

Pseudorandomised controlled study

An experimental comparison study in which subjects are allocated to treatment/intervention or control/placebo groups in a non-random way (such as alternate allocation, allocation by day of week, odd–even study numbers, etc).

Random error

The portion of variation in a measurement that is due to chance.

Randomised controlled trial

An experimental comparison study in which participants are allocated to treatment/intervention or control/placebo groups using a random mechanism (such as coin toss, random number table or computer-generated random numbers). Participants have an equal chance of being allocated to an intervention or control group and therefore allocation bias is eliminated.

Reference test (*see also* Index test)

A method, procedure or measurement that is widely regarded or accepted as being the best available (also known as a 'gold standard'). Often used to compare with a new method (index test).

Relative risk or risk ratio (RR)

Ratio of the rates of outcome in the treatment and control groups. This expresses the risk of the outcome in the treatment group relative to that in the control group.

Relative risk reduction (RRR)

The relative reduction in risk associated with an intervention or exposure. It is calculated as one minus the relative risk.

Secondary research

An academic review of primary research studies to gain new insights on a specific topic (such as a systematic review).

Selection bias

Error due to systematic differences in characteristics between those who are selected for study and those who are not. It invalidates conclusions and generalisations that might otherwise be drawn from such studies.

Systematic review (*see also* Secondary research)

The process of systematically locating, appraising and synthesising evidence from scientific studies in order to obtain a reliable overview.

Time series

A set of measurements taken over time. An interrupted time series is generated when a set of measurements is taken before the introduction of an intervention (or some other change in the system), followed by another set of measurements taken over time after the change.

Validity

Of a study: the degree to which the inferences drawn from the study are warranted when account is taken of the study methods, the representativeness of the study sample, and the nature of the population from which it is drawn (internal and external validity, applicability, generalisability).

Answers to quizzes and appraisals

Part 2, Step 1: The PICO principle — formulating questions (pages 26–35)

Interventions, Example 2: P = long-term smokers; I = acupuncture; C = (i) nothing or (ii) other interventions (eg nicotine replacement); O = quit smoking at 3–6 months

Note: As with many treatment questions, we may be interested in (i) whether it works at all, and so want a comparison with nothing (placebo) and then (ii) whether it works as well as or better than other treatments.

Question: In long-term smokers, does acupuncture, compared with other interventions, improve the chance of successfully quitting?

Interventions, Example 3: P = infants receiving immunisation; I = longer needles; C = shorter needles; O = local reactions

Question: In infants receiving immunisation injections, does needle length affect the rate of local reactions?

Aetiology and risk factors, Example 2: P = newborn babies; I = vitamin K injection; C = no vitamin K injection; O = childhood leukaemia

Question: In newborn babies, does a vitamin K injection increase the risk of childhood leukaemia?

Diagnosis, Example 2: P = elderly people ; I = whispered voice test; C = (i) no test or (ii) other test; O = hearing problem (eg as assessed by audiogram)

Note: Again, as for treatment we may be first interested in (i) whether the test is accurate at all (ie better than flipping a coin, which has a sensitivity and specificity of 50%!), and then (ii) whether it is at least as, or more, accurate than alternative surgery or clinic tests.

Question: In elderly people, does the whispered voice compared to other conventional tests give an accurate diagnosis of hearing problems?

Prognosis, Example 2: P = men with inguinal hernia; O = strangulation

Question: In men with a hernia, how likely is it that the hernia will strangulate?

Frequency or rate, Example 2: P = adults with lower back pain; O = more serious condition

Question: In adults with lower back pain, what is the frequency that the pain may reflect a more serious condition (such as tumour or infection)?

Phenomena, Example 2: P = patients on regular medications; O = methods to remember to take medications.

Part 2, Step 1: Formulate clinical questions (page 37)

Q1. **(b)** is clearly answerable (by cohort or randomised trial) and so is **(d)**, which can be answered first through qualitative research (the list of reasons) and then quantified

(c) is not directly answerable without specifying a set of possible treatments or comparisons; **(a)** is not answerable, but maybe we can discuss that over a drink?

Q2. **(a)** placebo (or 'nothing'), though if it does have an effect we may then be interested in how that compares with other alternatives; **(b)** low or normal homocysteine; **(c)** clear urine

Q3. **(a)** P = people with pneumonia; I = 3 days of antibiotics; C= 8 days of antibiotics (the standard); O = ? This is a treatment question, and hence we would like a randomised trial – as was done.

(b) P = normal population; I = (good?) personality and lifestyle; C = (poor?) personality and lifestyle; O = cardiovascular disease and cancer. This is initially an aetiology question (and hence a cohort is ideal) but if we then become interested in changing lifestyle or personality it becomes a treatment question and we'd like a randomised trial.

(c) P = newborn; I = one colour of vomit; C = other colours of vomit; O = intestinal obstruction

(d) P = people undergoing coronary artery bypass surgery; I = off-pump surgery; C = on-pump surgery; O = clinical, angiographic, neurocognitive and quality-of-life outcomes. This is a treatment question, and so a randomised trial is ideal, as was done.

Part 2, Step 2: Track down the best evidence

Abstract exercise (pages 43–47)

Abstract 1

Question	Answer	
1. What is the question (PICO) of the study?	P:	men (40–60 years)
	I:	high dietary intake of folate, vitamin B6, and vitamin B12
	C:	low dietary intake of …
	O:	acute coronary events
2. What is the purpose of the study?	Aetiology and risk factors	
3. Which primary study type would give the highest-quality evidence to answer the question?	RCT	
4. Which is the best study type that is also feasible?	RCT (see next abstract)	
5. What is the study type used?	Cohort study (prospective)	

Abstract 2

Question	Answer	
1. What is the question (PICO) of the study?	P:	adults (>55 years) with vascular disease or diabetes
	I:	folate, vitamin B6, and vitamin B12 supplements
	C:	no supplements
	O:	death from cardiovascular causes, myocardial infarction and stroke
2. What is the purpose of the study?	Intervention (folate supplementation)	
3. Which primary study type would give the highest-quality evidence to answer the question?	RCT	
4. Which is the best study type that is also feasible?	RCT	
5. What is the study type used?	RCT	

Abstract 3

Question	Answer	
1. What is the question (PICO) of the study?	P:	adults (community-based)
	I:	
	C:	
	O:	snoring, asthma and sleep complaints
2. What is the purpose of the study?	Frequency	
3. Which primary study type would give the highest-quality evidence to answer the question?	Cross-sectional survey	
4. Which is the best study type that is also feasible?	Cross-sectional survey	
5. What is the study type used?	Cross-sectional survey	

Abstract 4

Question	Answer	
1. What is the question (PICO) of the study?	P:	infants
	I:	abnormal stool colour
	C:	normal stool colour
	O:	diagnosis of biliary atresia
2. What is the purpose of the study?	Diagnosis	
3. Which primary study type would give the highest-quality evidence to answer the question?	Diagnostic cross-sectional study	
4. Which is the best study type that is also feasible?	Diagnostic cross-sectional study	
5. What is the study type used?	Diagnostic cross-sectional study (actually a very short-term follow-up)	

Abstract 5

Question	Answer	
1. What is the question (PICO) of the study?	P:	children diagnosed with headaches
	I:	
	C:	
	O:	frequency and type of headaches in adulthood
2. What is the purpose of the study?	Prognosis	
3. Which primary study type would give the highest-quality evidence to answer the question?	Prospective cohort study	
4. Which is the best study type that is also feasible?	Prospective cohort study	
5. What is the study type used?	Prospective cohort study	

Part 2, Step 2: Track down the best evidence (pages 68–69)

Q1. 1. C 2. D 3. E 4. A

Q2. 1. A 2. D 3. G 4. J 5. E 6. C 7. L 8. K

Q3.

A. NO, a correct formulation is

(elderly OR old) AND prevent* AND (fall OR fracture)

B. NO, a correct formulation is

ginkgo AND ((blood AND pressure) OR hypertension)

Part 2, Step 3: Critically appraise the evidence (page 131)

Q1. All these are important, but the most important is **(e)** the concealed randomisation list followed by **(d)** the blinding for non-objective measurements. For a discussion of the evidence for this see: Schulz KF, Chalmers I, Hayes RJ, Altman DG (1995). Empirical evidence of bias. Dimensions of methodological quality associated with estimates of treatment effects in controlled trials. JAMA 273(5):408–412.

Q2. Again all these are are important, but the most important are firstly **(e)** the quality of the included studies (it's not whether they were appraised, but whether you can tell that they are sufficiently high quality) and secondly **(c)** the quality of the search — did they find most studies and/ or do an analysis of publication bias? And **(b)** were there clear inclusion/ exclusion criteria so that they were not selecting on the basis of results but on the basis of eligibility (the inclusion criteria will have both PICO and RAMMbo elements)?

Part 2, Step 4: Apply the evidence (pages 139–140)

Q1. The ARR is 13%–9%=4%, and hence the NNT is 1/0.04 = 25 patients need to be treated to prevent one death.

Q2. Since the patient's expected event rate is one-third (ie 3%) and the relative risk reduction is the same, then the ARR is also one-third of the trial's ARR, that is 4/3% or 1.33%, and hence the NNT is 75.

Q3. **(a)** The strengths are that it is a randomised trial, it is of moderate size (600 patients), and there is single blinding (of outcome assessors). Weaknesses are the single blinding (but it's not possible to double blind this) and the short follow-up (or the total person time), particularly given the small number of events (16 cardiac deaths in the control group).

(b) The risk ratio of 0.27 means the relative risk of an event in the treatment group was 27% of that in the risk in the control group, that is, a reduction in risk of 73%.

(c) The control event rate (CER) is 16+17/303 = 11% and the experimental event rate (EER) is 8/302 = 3%, hence the ARR is 8%, and the NNT is 1/0.08 = 12.

(d) The study stopped early, and has not been replicated, so the positive effect may be an overestimate. However, it might be reasonable to say that the evidence is not definitive, but the Mediterranean diet plus alpha-linolenic acid (as margarine) seems to reduce risk, so if she is happy with such a diet it seems medically sensible.

Part 3: Critical appraisal of a prognostic study – the VT recurrence study (pages 144–151)

Q1. What is the PICO of the VT study?

P = patients over 18 who had been treated for at least 3 months with anticoagulation after a deep vein thrombosis (I = men C = women); O = recurrence of deep vein thrombosis. (The I and C are in brackets as their main question was probably the PO of recurrence; but an analysis of predictors revealed the male-female difference.)

Q2. How well was the study done?

Recruitment: All the patients were from 4 thrombosis centres in Vienna. It is useful to draw the flowchart of these patients:

2795 attended with 1945 excluded (450 previous DVT, etc)

850 remained — a further 24 excluded with specific deficiencies

826 started follow-up (ie only about 1/3 of all DVT cases).

Adjustment: Table 1 shows both the univariate (single factor) and multivariate (multiple factor) analyses. These show similar results, with an important exception being age, which becomes non-significant when other factors are adjusted for — that is, these other factors appear to 'explain' the impact of age.

Maintenance: 189 'left' the study — 125 who required antithrombotic treatment for reasons other than DVT and 40 with cancer or pregnancy; and 24 were lost to follow-up. That latter figure (24/826 = 3%) is acceptable.

Measurement: Made using venography (definition given) and assessed by a committee blinded to the presence of risk factors.

Q3. What do the results mean?

See Figure 1 in the paper.

(1) The risk of recurrence in men at 1 year is about 10% and at five years about 30%. (2) The 3-year risk in men is about 21% and in women about 7%. This is an absolute difference of 21−7 = 14%. The relative risk of recurrence is 21/7 = 3.0. Note that we could also express this as the relative risk of non-recurrence, which would be 79/93 = 0.85. (3) 20% (1 in 5) men have had a recurrence a bit before 3 years — about 2 years and 9 months.

Overall this is a good-quality study, but we need to be cautious about generalising to other groups and be aware that the results apply to only about one-third of patients (who don't have the exclusion factors). The recurrence rates may be lower in the group excluded with trauma or surgery, and higher in those with previous recurrence.

Part 3: Critical appraisal of a study of diagnostic test accuracy – the whispered voice test (pages 162–168)

Q1. What is the PICO of the whispered voice test study?

P= patients attending with aural symptoms; I (index test) = whispered voice test; C = Pat-225, Audioscope-3, Micromate-304; O = the outcome is hearing loss (as assessed by an audiogram)

Q2. How well was the study done?

Recruitment: All patients were attending an outpatient ENT department — the use of all patients is good; but the spectrum of illness will depend on the referral pattern to this clinic. Patients are over 55 years, but no other details are given.

Allocation: The index and reference tests were applied independently of each other.

Maintenance: There is no statement about whether some patients missed having the tests or the audiogram, but as this is a 'captive' group maintenance is likely to have been high.

Measurements: The outcome is measured by audiogram which is relatively, but not completely, objective. It is not stated who did the audiogram and whether they knew the whispered voice result so we cannot assume blinding.

Q3. What do the results mean?

1. See table below. The sensitivity was 66/73 = 90% and the specificity was 41/51 = 80%. The post-test probability after a positive (abnormal) result is 66/76 = 88% and the post-test probability after a negative (normal) result is 7/48 = 15%.

	Abnormal audiogram	Normal audiogram	Total
Abnormal WVT	66	10	76
Normal WVT	7	41	48
Total	73	51	124

2. The whispered voice test was compared to 3 other tests and was clearly better than the Madsen Part 225, but less sensitive than the audioscope. We could also compare all tests to a coin flip which has a sensitivity of 50% and a specificity of 50%, so it is clearly (much) better than chance.

Overall the paper is incompletely reported, so the generalisation in particular is difficult. In this setting it appears to perform well but the patients here may have more severe aural problems, and the test may not be as good in primary care settings. The pre-test chance of hearing problems was very high (over half) and this is likely to be lower elsewhere. A nice feature of the paper was the use of several examiners which demonstrated the variation in accuracy in different hands.

Endpiece

We hope this book has helped you learn how to keep up to date with current knowledge to look after your patients, and work with others to achieve this goal.

Although we have tried to correct flaws in this new edition, we recognise that there are probably still many shortcomings and suboptimal examples. If you notice ways of improving the book, please feel free to contact us (our email addresses are below). We would love to hear from you if you have any comments — positive or less positive — and we will incorporate improvements (suitably acknowledged of course) in a 3rd edition of the workbook.

We have also prepared some teaching slides from the contents of the workbook, which you can access at the following website:

http://www.cebm.net/EBP-workbook

Finally, we hope this book stimulates you to find the evidence to help with good patient care. We also think that this book can contribute to making patient care, that most satisfying responsibility, even more fun!

Paul Glasziou (paul.glasziou@dphpc.ox.ac.uk)

Chris Del Mar (CDelMar@bond.edu.au)

Janet Salisbury (janet.salisbury@biotext.com.au)

Index

Page numbers in *italics* represent figures, those in **bold** represent tables.